T0383786

Intraoperative Neurophysiological Monitoring in Hemifacial Spasm

Sang-Ku Park
Byung-Euk Joo • Kwan Park

Intraoperative Neurophysiological Monitoring in Hemifacial Spasm

A Practical Guide

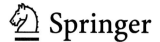 Springer

Sang-Ku Park
Department of Neurosurgery
Konkuk University Medical Center
Seoul
Korea (Republic of)

Byung-Euk Joo
Department of Neurology
Soonchunhyang University Hospital
Seoul
Korea (Republic of)

Kwan Park
Department of Neurosurgery
Konkuk University Medical Center
Seoul
Korea (Republic of)

ISBN 978-981-16-1326-5   ISBN 978-981-16-1327-2   (eBook)
https://doi.org/10.1007/978-981-16-1327-2

This Springer imprint is published by the registered company Springer Nature Singapore Pte Ltd.
The registered company address is: 152 Beach Road, #21-01/04 Gateway East, Singapore
189721, Singapore

'The contents covered in this book are data measured with real-time BAEPs and new method LSR. The test method newly developed by the authors was able to improve efficiency and achieve shorter test time than the existing method.'

Preface

This book is a comprehensive and up-to-date intraoperative neurophysiological monitoring guide to hemifacial spasm, one of the very few neuromuscular disorders that can be treated surgically.

All aspects are covered, including BAEP change, lateral spread response, free-running EMG and facial MEP, blink reflex and F wave, complications, prognosis, and patterns of hearing loss during surgery.

Dr. Kwan Park has performed microvascular decompression surgery, the treatment of choice, in more than 4500 hemifacial spasm patients at Samsung Medical Center in Seoul, Korea. And medical technologist Sang ku Park has performed neurological tests in all surgeries. In addition, many new test methods were proposed, contributing to higher test reliability. In particular, Dr. Byung-EukJoo explains detailed and complete neuro-monitoring based on his experience in clinical neurophysiology.

This book draws together the many scientific contributions of neurosurgeon Dr. Kwan Park, medical technologist Sang ku Park, and neurophysiologist Dr. Byung-EukJoo and offers the very latest insights into management of the condition.

This book is all about the various situations that occur during surgery, and the causes and solutions of the situations are explained in an easy language. In addition, the results of each test and their association with the postoperative prognosis are comprehensively explained.

It will be an excellent guide for young neurosurgeons, neurological monitoring technologists, and neurological interpreters.

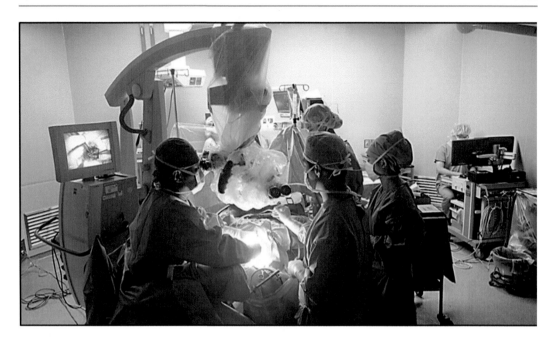

Contents

Principles of Intraoperative Neurophysiological Monitoring During MVD for HFS

1.1 Brainstem Auditory Evoked Potentials (BAEPs)

1.1.1 Introduction

A transient auditory stimulus can evoke a complex series of auditory evoked potentials lasting for hundreds of milliseconds. (Fig. 1.1) The middle-latency and long-latency auditory evoked potentials are markedly attenuated by surgical anesthesia, so these potentials are not useful for intraoperative neurophysiologic monitoring (INM) of the integrity of the auditory pathways. The short-latency auditory evoked potentials, with latencies of less than 10 milliseconds in normal unanesthetized adult subjects, are relatively unaf-fected by surgical anesthesia and are also easy record with waveforms that are consistent across subjects, so these potentials are the most useful for INM. Though they are not entirely generated in the brainstem, they are most often referred to as "brainstem auditory evoked potentials".

1.1.2 Waveforms

BAEPs are recorded between the vertex (electrode location Cz of the international 10–20 system for electrode placement) and the earlobe or mastoid ipsilateral to the stimulated ear (Ai); other recording channels may also be useful those involving the contralateral earlobe or mastoid.

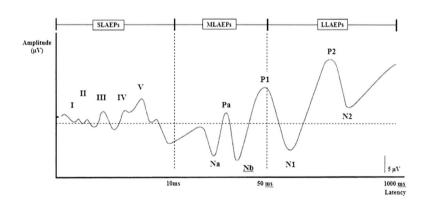

Fig. 1.1 Auditory evoked potentials. *SLAEPs* short-latency auditory evoked potentials, *MLAEPs* middle-latency auditory evoked potentials, *LLAEPs*, long-latency auditory evoked potentials

S.-K. Park et al., *Intraoperative Neurophysiological Monitoring in Hemifacial Spasm*, https://doi.org/10.1007/978-981-16-1327-2_1

Fig. 1.2 Brainstem auditory evoked potentials

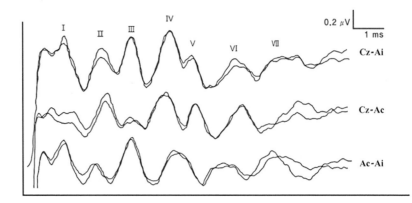

Positivity at the vertex is usually represented as an upward deflection, and the upward-going peaks are labeled with Roman numerals. (Fig. 1.2) Wave I is often followed by The BAEPs waveform typically begins with an electrical stimulus artifact that is synchronous with stimulus production at the transducer [1]. Wave I is the first major upgoing peak of the Cz–Ai waveform. The cochlear microphonic may be visible as a separate peak preceding wave I, but can be distinguished by reversing the stimulus polarity, which will reverse the polarity of the cochlear microphonic. Wave I may show a latency shift, but will not reverse polarity with this maneuver. Wave II is typically the first major upward deflection in the Cz–Ac waveform, and is similar in amplitude between the Cz–Ai and Cz–Ac waveforms. However, it is small and difficult to identify in some normal subjects. A substantial wave III is usually present in both the Cz–Ai and Cz–Ac channels but is smaller in the latter. A bifid wave III, or a very small wave III in the presence of a clear wave V at normal latency, is a normal variant waveform. The IV–V complex is often the most prominent component in the BAEPs waveform and is usually followed by a large negative deflection (VN or the slow negativity) that lasts several milliseconds and brings the waveform to a point below the pre-stimulus baseline. The morphology of the IV–V complex varies from one subject to another subject, and may differ between the two ears in the same person. There may be a smoothly fused waveform, two separate peaks, or one of the peaks visible as an inflection on the rising or falling phase of the other. If the latency of wave V cannot be accurately measured in the Cz–Ai waveform,

then it can be measured in the Cz–Ac waveform, where waves IV and V are more separated. However, this latency measurement should be compared with normative data that were recorded in a Cz–Ac channel. The stimulus parameters can be modified to help identify or confirm the identification of wave V. Wave V is the BAEPs component most resistant to the effects of decreasing stimulus intensity or increasing stimulus rate. If either of these stimulus modifications is performed progressively until only one component remains, that peak can be identified as wave V and then traced back through the series of waveforms to identify wave V in the BAEPs recorded with the standard stimulus.

1.1.3 Anatomical Generators

Wave I is generated in the most distal portion (cochlear end) of the auditory nerve and arises from the first volley of action potentials in the nerve, [2] corresponding to the N1 component of the eighth nerve CAP in the ECochG. Its origin in the most distal portion of the nerve is demonstrated by its occasional persistence after section of the auditory nerve during resection of eighth nerve tumors. Initial generator models for BAEPs proposed a single anatomical generator for each peak, but it has subsequently been shown that the BAEPs peaks after wave I are the composites of contributions from multiple generators, 8 as originally proposed by Jewett and Williston. In many cases, however, clinical–pathological correlations suggest predominant contributions to a component from a specific anatomical area. In the single anatomic generator models, wave II is usually associated with the cochlear nucleus. Activity at the level of the cochlear nucleus, driven by the first auditory nerve volley, does contribute to wave II. However, the second volley in the distal auditory nerve, the N2 component of the eighth nerve CAP, occurs at the same time as this, and also contributes to the scalp-recorded wave II. Thus, wave II can persist when the proximal eighth nerve has been destroyed. Wave III predominantly reflects activity in auditory system neurons in the caudal pontine tegmentum, including the region of the superior olivary complex, though a contribution from continued activity at the level of the cochlear nucleus cannot be ruled out. Because ascending projections from the cochlear nucleus are bilateral, wave III may receive contributions from brainstem auditory structures both ipsilateral and contralateral to the stimulated ear. In patients with asymmetrical or unilateral brainstem lesions of the lower pons, wave III abnormalities are usually most pronounced after stimulation of the ear ipsilateral to the lesion. Brainstem auditory evoked potential abnormalities in patients with unilateral auditory nerve dysfunction will be manifested after stimulation of the ipsilateral ear, of course. The anatomical generators of waves IV and V are most likely in close anatomical proximity or overlapping, because they are usually either both affected or both unaffected by brainstem lesions, although there are exceptions. Wave IV seems to reflect activity predominantly in ascending auditory fibers within the dorsal and rostral pons, just caudal to the inferior colliculus, whereas wave V predominantly reflects activity at the level of the inferior colliculus, perhaps including activity in the rostral portion of the lateral lemniscus because it terminates in the inferior colliculus. As is the case with wave III, wave V abnormalities due to unilateral brainstem lesions are usually most pronounced after stimulation of the ear ipsilateral to the lesion, although there are exceptions. While waves VI and VII may in part reflect activity in more rostral structures such as the medial geniculate nucleus, they also receive contributions from activity in the inferior colliculus. The latter generator may cause persistence of these waves in patients with auditory pathway damage rostral to the inferior colliculus. In addition, these components are absent in some normal subjects. Therefore, BAEPs cannot be used to assess or monitor the auditory pathways rostral to the mesencephalon. The anatomic generators of BAEPs are shown in Fig. 1.3.

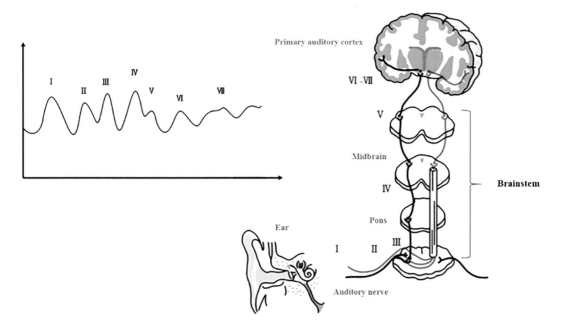

Fig. 1.3 Anatomical generator of brainstem auditory evoked potentials

1.2   Lateral Spread Response

Lateral spread response (LSR) is the unique triggered electromyography (EMG) response for hemifacial spasm (HFS). In HFS, an abnormal spread response called as LSR, is elicited by stimulation of the facial nerve branch and is recorded from facial muscles innervated by another branch (Fig. 1.4). In 1985, Møller and Jannetta showed that in the HFS, due to the hyperexcitability of the facial nerve, the stimulation of one branch of facial nerve activates facial muscles innervated by another branch producing abnormal muscle responses. The LSR can be recorded from one muscle innervated by the superior branch of the facial nerve when the inferior branch is stimulated or vice versa. The LSR has been related to ephaptic transmission but it was Møller et al. who demonstrated that the abnormal responses are due to the facial motor nucleus hyperactivity. Due to the fact that LSR disappears instantly in most of the patients when the offending vessel is moved off the facial nerve, LSR have been considered as a useful intraoperative tool to ensure the adequate decompression of the facial nerve during MVD for HFS [3, 4]. Numerous studies have demonstrated a positive correlation between the intraoperative disappearance of LSR and favorable outcome in patients undergoing MVD for HFS; therefore,

LSR has been used as an indicator of complete facial nerve decompression. The LSR usually disappears after microvascular decompression in patients with HFS, with the nerve considered to be adequately decompressed. However, controversial findings, such as LSR absence before MVD or LSR persistence after MVD, have been reported. Furthermore, several studies suggested that residual LSR after MVD was not related to long-term outcome of HFS; conversely, other studies concluded that repeated MVD was necessary because residual LSR indicates insufficient decompression. Therefore, the practical value of LSR disappearance as an indicator of adequate decompression remains controversial.

1.3   Free-running EMG

Free-running EMG (Fr EMG) provides information regarding mechanical or thermal facial nerve injury. Nerve injury is manifested as sustained, high-frequency neurotonic discharges in facial nerve EMG. If this activity is detected, the neurophysiologist can provide immediate feedback to the neurosurgeon to allow operative maneuver changes to avoid nerve injury. Fr EMG activity in muscles innervated by the facial nerve was mainly studied in cerebellopontine angle surgery.

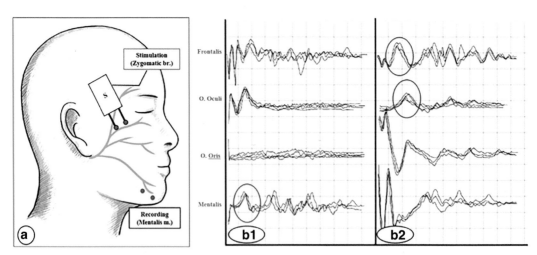

Fig. 1.4 Lateral spread response. (**a**): When stimulating the temporal or zygomatic branch of the facial nerve, LSR is recorded from mentalis or orbicularis oris muscles, that innervated by another branch of facial nerve. (**b**): In **b-1**, LSR is recorded form mentalis muscle by sitmulation of zygmatic branch of facial nerve. In **b-2**, LSR is seen form frontalis and orbicularis oculi muscles by stimulation of buccal branch of facial nerve. LSR is marked with a red circle

Romstöck et al. proposed a classification system for the patterns of facial nerve Fr EMG by separating spikes, bursts, and three different kinds of train-patterns with respect to waveform and frequency characteristics [5]. The term "train" was introduced for sustained periodic EMG activity that lasts for seconds. Three typical train patterns with specific rhythmic features were observed. The A-train is the most important of these patterns. This train is a distinct EMG waveform of sinusoidal pattern that has maximum amplitudes ranging from 100 to 200 μV, and a frequency up to 210 Hz. Their duration varies between milliseconds and several seconds. They can display as a single long pattern, or as a salvo of short A-trains. The occurrence of A-trains was shown to be associated with postoperative facial palsy with high sensitivity (86%) and specificity (89%) during cerebellopontine angle tumor surgeries. In patients with HFS, irregular Fr EMG activity can be spontaneously elicited during MVD, especially when saline is injected onto the facial nerve. When the ratio of post-MVD to pre-MVD Fr EMG activity was calculated to assess Fr EMG activity, Fr EMG activity ratios of $\geq$50% were reported to be associated with a greater likelihood of a residual LSR in patients with HFS.

1.4   Others (Facial Motor Evoked Potentials, Blink Reflex, Facial F-wave)

1.4.1   Facial Motor Evoked Potentials

Although uncommonly performed, myogenic facial motor evoked potentials (facial MEP) elicited through transcranial electric stimulation can be used to monitor the functional integrity of the FMN during MVD surgery. Facial MEP monitoring in patients with HFS has remarkable characteristics due to hyperexcitability of the FMN. Also, the stimulation threshold for eliciting a facial MEP response has been observed to increase after successful decompression of the facial nerve. Therefore, the facial MEP threshold before and after MVD can be used as an indicator of a successful MVD.

1.4.2   Blink Reflex Test

Trigeminal) and facial nerve, along with their connections in the pons and medullar, can be assessed electrically with the blink reflex (Fig. 1.5). The blink reflex is essentially the electrical correlated of the clinically evoked corneal reflex. The blink reflex is a true reflex, with a sensory afferent limb, intervening synapses, and a motor efferent. Blink reflexes are useful in detecting abnormalities anywhere along the reflex arc, including peripheral and central pathways. The afferent limb of the blink reflex is mediated by sensory fibers of the supraorbital branch of the ophthalmic division of the trigeminal nerve and the efferent limb by motor fibers of the facial nerve. Just as with the corneal reflex, ipsilateral electrical stimulation of the supraoptic branch of the trigeminal nerve elicits a facial nerve (eye blink) response bilaterally. Stimulation of the ipsilateral supraorbital nerve results in an afferent volley along the trigeminal nerve to both the main sensory nucleus of trigeminal nerve (mid-pons) and the nucleus of the spinal tract of trigeminal nerve (lower pons and medulla) in the brainstem. Through a series of interneurons in the pons and lateral medullar, the nerve impulse next reaches the ipsilateral and contralateral facial nuclei, from which the efferent signal travels along the facial nerve bilaterally.

The blink reflex has two components: an early R1 and a late R2 response. R1 response is evoked ipsilaterally to stimulation site, whereas R2 response is evoked bilaterally. R1 response is thought to represent the disynaptic reflex pathway between the main sensory nucleus of V in the mid pons and the ipsilateral facial nucleus in the lower pontine tegmentum. R2 responses are mediated by a multisynaptic pathway between the nucleus of the spinal tract of V in the ipsilateral pons and medulla and interneurons forming connections to the ipsilateral and contralateral facial nuclei. To investigate the pathophysiology for HFS, blink reflex test was performed in the previous many studies. For example, Eekhof et al. reported that the HFS patients had a significantly higher amplitude of R1 and R2 responses in the orbicularis oris as compared with normal controls [6]. Valls-Sole et al. also showed that the area of R1 and R2 responses was greater on the

a

b

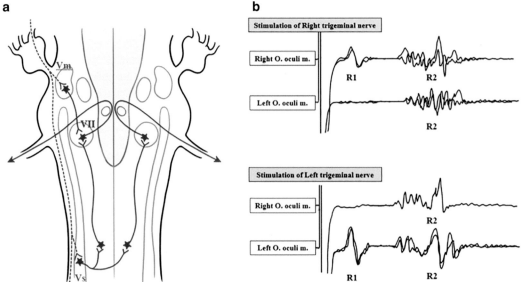

Fig. 1.5 Anatomy and waveforms of the blink reflex. (**a**): The afferent limb of the blink reflex is mediated by sensory fibers of the supraorbital branch of the ophthalmic division of the trigeminal nerve, which synapses with both the main sensory nucleus (Vm) in the midpons and the nucleus of the spinal tract (Vs) in the medulla. The earlier R1 response is mediated by a disynaptic connection between the Vm nucleus and the ipsilateral facial motor nucleus (VII). The later R2 response are mediated by multisynaptic pathway between the Vs nucleus and both ipsilateral and contralateral facial nucleus (VII). (**b**). By stimulation of right trigeminal nerve, earlier R1 responses is recorded on ipsilateral right orbicularis oculi muscle, later R2 responses are obtained on ipsilateral and contralateral orbicularis oculi muscles

symptomatic side in the patients with HFS as compared with the asymptomatic side and normal controls [7]. In addition, the authors reported a bilaterally enhanced recovery of the blink reflex on R2 responses in the HFS patients by performing the paired-stimulus blink reflex test and concluded that interneurons mediating the brainstem reflex pathway were hyperexcitable. Larger blink reflex responses on the symptomatic side in HFS have been observed in different groups.

1.4.3   Facial F-wave Study

The facial F-wave represents the backfiring of the facial motor neurons after being activated antidromically. F-wave activity was shown to be an index of motor neuron excitability. F-wave persistence appearance was reported in patients with HFS and found to decrease after adequate MVD, albeit with delay as long as 2 years. It is possible to record changes in elicitability of the facial F-wave during MVD. Immediate changes in hyperexcitability of the FMN can be observed by monitoring changes in F-wave elicitability. Facial F-waves can

be obtained from the mentalis muscle by stimulating the mandibular branch of the facial nerve.

References

1. Legatt AD. Electrophysiology of cranial nerve testing: auditory nerve. J Clin Neurophysiol. 2018;35(1):25–38.
2. Legatt AD, Arezzo JC, Vaughan HG Jr. The anatomic and physiologic bases of brain stem auditory evoked potentials. Neurol Clin. 1988;6(4):681–704.
3. Møller AR, Jannetta PJ. Microvascular decompression in hemifacial spasm: intraoperative electrophysiological observations. Neurosurgery. 1985;16:612–8.
4. Moller AR, Jannetta PJ. Monitoring facial EMG responses during microvascular decompression operations for hemifacial spasm. J Neurosurg. 1987;66(5):681–5.
5. Romstöck J, Strauss C, Fahlbusch R. Continuous electromyography monitoring of motor cranial nerves during cerebellopontine angle surgery. J Neurosurg. 2000;93(4):586–93.
6. Eekhof JL, Aramideh M, Speelman JD, Devriese PP. Ongerboer De Visser BW. Blink reflexes and lateral spreading in patients with synkinesia after Bell's palsy and in hemifacial spasm. Eur Neurol. 2000;43(3):141–6.
7. Valls-Sole J, Tolosa ES. Blink reflex excitability cycle in hemifacial spasm. Neurology. 1989;39(8):1061–6.

Methods of Intraoperative Neurophysiological Monitoring for Microvascular Decompression

2

2.1 Importance of Real-Time BAEPs Monitoring During INM

During surgery we commonly experience the following phenomena. The BAEPs wave V latency was observed to be prolonged to less than 1 ms, and the amplitude was also slightly decreased to less than 50% during surgery. In addition, after completing the averaging time where a slight change in waveform was observed, we must have experienced the case where all lost waveforms were suddenly measured after the next test. In this case of BAEPs loss, the brain retractor was immediately removed, and the waveform waited for recovery, but the waveform did not recover until the operation was completed, and the patient may have experienced HL after surgery. Through this experience, we have thought that the BAEPs wave change for the cochlear nerve function is very sensitive, so it is judged to alarm for surgeon that it is a dangerous state even if a very minute change occurs for the BAEPs wave change.

However, in some surgery, BAEPs wave V latency is observed to be extended by more than 1 ms, but it is maintained without any further change in the waveform, and it is commonly observed when it recovers to a normal waveform at the end of the surgery. In another surgery, the amplitude decreased by more than 50% and then recovered to normal. All of these patients had normal hearing after surgery. In particular, we know from experience that when the brain retractor is pulled severely in the main procedure, the change of the BAEPs waveform is not immediately observed, but the change of the BAEPs waveform occurs after the retraction continues for a long time.

Taken together, we concluded that the change in BAEPs waveform for cochlear nerve injury does not occur immediately. Looking at the settings generally used, if the averaging time is set to 1000 and the stimulation rate is set to 10 Hz, it takes 100 seconds. We thought that 100 seconds was too long, and we reduced the averaging time to make the BAEPs test faster. Observing the BAEPs waveform, the waveform shakes like a wave until the averaging time 100 to 200 times, and it does not have a specific shape. However, from no. 300 times, the shape of a stable waveform gradually began to be established, and from no. 400, very stable and specific waves I, III, and V were observed. And even if the averaging time is continued and test is performed up to 2000 times, there is no significant difference, and the shape of the averaging time 400 is maintained. So we decided to shorten the averaging time to 400 times. Stimulation rate was tested in various ways from 10 Hz to 100 Hz. Then, waveforms were formed at all Hz, and external artifacts were sometimes reflected in the waveform too quickly above 50 Hz, so we chose the 40 Hz band less than 50 Hz. So, we set up fast stimulation that tests in 9.1 seconds at 400 times averaging time and 43.9 Hz stimulation rate. We named this test method real-time BAEPs [1] (Fig. 2.1).

These days, because the sampling rate of intraoperative neurophysiological monitoring machines is very high, most of the equipments that have the ability to analyze one second are more than 20,000 ~ 65,000 Hz, so it is possible to perform a test that can see the results within 10 seconds.

While testing with real-time BAEPs, we observed new phenomena that we have not experienced so far, and we learned three major new features as follows.

First, BAEPs wave V latency is quite often extended gradually from dura open. To explain in detail, the wave V latency extends very slowly and continuously. Even if there is no particular abnormality, it is often extended to less than 1 ms and then recovered. When the cochlear nerve was affected a little more due

to the brain retractor, it was extended to 2 ms and then recovered, and in some cases, it was extended to 3 ms and then recovered (Fig. 2.2). Second, the wave V amplitude changes even within 9.1 seconds. Unlike the change in latency, it shows a pattern in which a sharp decrease is observed. In the case of severe damage, it was also experienced that it was lost in 9.1 seconds.

Third, it always shows a pattern in which the wave V latency extension occurs first and then the amplitude change occurs. In the case of only prolonged wave V latency, there was no change in hearing after surgery, and when the decrease in amplitude is observed after prolonged wave V latency, there are occasional changes in hearing after surgery. There was a case where it was not possible to prevent the loss of amplitude, which rapidly decreased even if the test was performed in 9.1 seconds with the real-time BAEPs method. Even if the

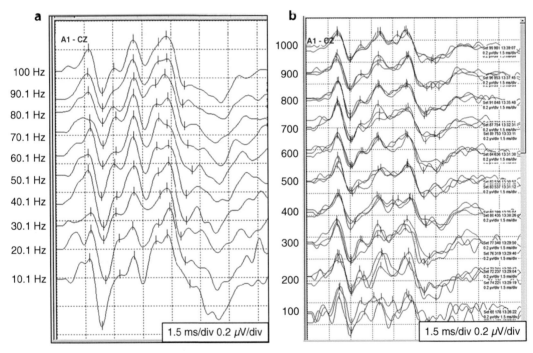

Fig. 2.1 (a) Waveform change according to stimulation rate (with averaging of 1000 trials). (b) Averaging trials (with 43.9 Hz/sec stimulation rate) from IOM of BAEPs. Although the waveform was formed from 10 Hz to 100 Hz, the faster the test above 50 Hz, the more the waveform was affected by the surgical operation. Thus,

when the test was performed at a speed of about 40 Hz, stable waveforms were not affected by the surgical operation. Reproducibility was enough about 400 times to achieve the same effect as 1000 times of averaging time. (These results are from BE Joo et al. J Neurosurg 2016 Nov;125(5):1061–1067)

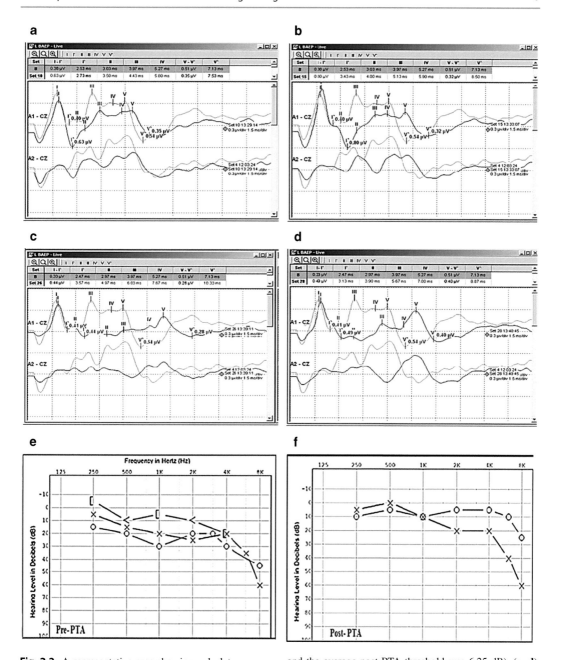

Fig. 2.2 A representative case showing only latency prolongation (≥1 ms) without a significant change in amplitude (the latency of wave V was delayed by 3.20 ms from 7.13 to 10.33 ms with a minimal decrease in the amplitude). The patient in this example did not experience postoperative hearing loss. (The average pre-PTA threshold was 22.5 dB, and the average post-PTA threshold was 6.25 dB). (**a–d**) The INM of BAEPs during MVD surgery (green line = baseline of wave V; black line = wave V showing maximal prolongation in latency), (**e**) pre operative pure tone audiometry (**f**) pure tone audiometry of the patients obtained prior to surgery and 7 days postoperatively

waveform was rapidly lost in 9.1 seconds during surgery, cochlear nerve damage was detected quickly, and if surgical measures were taken, no further damage was caused.

BAEPs warning criteria exist slightly differently according to surgeon's experience. There is a paper on the importance of changing BAEPs wave V latency [2–4]. There are papers such as wave V latency 0.4 ms, 0.6 ms, and 1 ms [5, 6]. This may be due to a loss of waveform in the next BAEPs test after showing an extension of the wave V latency of 0.4 ms to 1 ms, or the patient's hearing impairment after surgery. Unlike this, there is also a paper that the change in wave V amplitude is important [7–10]. An amplitude that changes in 9.1 seconds can never be discriminated by a waveform with a test time of 100 seconds or more. For example, up to 900 times were normal, and the cochlear nerve was damaged at the remaining 100 times averaging time, but the shape of the waveform could not be seriously changed because it was a normal wave up to 900 times. So, the amplitude that shows a change that decreases rapidly in a short time is inevitably reflected as a very small change in waveform in the entire averaging time, so even if it is measured as if the amplitude decreases by 50%, it may be a dangerous state.

Latency shows a steady change gradually, so even with a long averaging time of 1000 tests, the change in the waveform is clearly observed rather than the amplitude. Therefore, it can be seen that it is natural that the warning criteria were set mainly for latency in the past.

The criteria widely known as BAEPs warning criteria are the latency of wave V, delayed by 1 ms, and amplitude decreased by 50% [11, 12]. If BAEPs are being tested in a way that takes more than 100 seconds, these criteria should be applied to intraoperative monitoring. However, if you know that the amplitude can decrease rapidly within 10 seconds, you will need to do a test to discern this change in amplitude.

Real-time BAEPs test is a fast stimulation method and helps a lot in discriminating whether or not the actual cochlear nerve is damaged. Stimulation rate is 43.9 Hz, averaging time is 400, it is not necessary to adhere to the standard, and it is okay to perform faster stimulation rate. This criterion is only the best way we have found. You should try to find the optimal settings that are slightly different for different devices and to perform the fastest test.

If you quickly observe the waveform change by performing a real-time BAEPs test, you can observe the characteristic change patterns of waves I, III, and V.

2.1.1 Characteristic Patterns of Wave I

- As wave II disappears, it is observed very often as if I-I' became larger. This happens when the cochlear nerve is very weakly damaged.
- It is well observed that wave I itself is delayed.
- When BAEPs loss occurs, it is divided into a case where wave I exists and a case where all waveforms are lost. (Detailed in Chap. 3)

2.1.2 Characteristic Patterns of Wave III

- In many cases, wave III delayed even with slight influence. It is possible to clearly identify whether wave III delay occurs due to an extension from wave I or only wave III delayed, so that the degree of damage to the cochlear nerve can be clearly identified.
- Wave III loss is observed too often. However, this wave III loss is not significantly related to postoperative hearing loss.

2.1.3 Characteristic Patterns of Wave V

- Latency extension can be observed only by dura open, and latency delayed continues to progress slowly. In some cases, extension is observed even up to 3 ms, and it recovers to normal after the main procedure.
- The amplitude rapidly decreases by more than 50% within 10 seconds. Some more severe damage may be lost within 10 seconds. Most of the lost waveforms recover during surgery, but in many cases, HL occurs after surgery when surgery is terminated in a lost state. When the amplitude was reduced by 50%, it was found that the waveform is often lost if the operation is continued. So, it is very important that we do not proceed with the surgery when the wave V amplitude is reduced by 50% and proceed after the waveform is recov-

ered. We consider the 50% reduction in wave V amplitude as the wave reversible point.

2.2 BAEPs Monitoring

The origin of each waveform is as follows: the I wave is the distal portion of the cochlear nerve; the II wave is the frequency, intensity, and phase of the wave sound originating from the proximal portion of the cochlear nerve. It plays a role of transferring information about the phase. Wave III performs the information processing of time and frequency and the control role of sending the wave neuron information from the cochlear nucleus to the appropriate part of the auditory nerve system. The wave IV functions to analyze the difference in the time difference and the intensity of the wave generated in the superior olivary complex. Therefore, it plays an important role in locating the sound source. Wave V is the most important path of the auditory system in the lateral lemniscus. It responds sensitively to the change of the negative stimulus by time and stimulus size. Wave VI and wave VII occur in the inferior colliculus, which also deal with auditory and somatosensory information. Wave VI and wave VII are not all observed, so they are generally excluded from the waveform evaluation [13].

When real-time BAEPs are tested, the shape of the waveform reflects a more practical cochlear nerve function than the conventional method. So, sometimes the shape of the waveform is smooth and not pretty. In particular, in the case of a flat wave due to the loss of the waveform, it is often observed that the waveform is slightly wrinkled. So, there may be a case of misunderstanding as if the waveform is weakly formed. In other words, even though the waveform is lost, an error of expression such as a 90% reduction in the waveform can be made. So, if it has reproducibility when inspected more than three times, it is recognized as a waveform; otherwise it should not be recognized as a waveform. In this case, if you observe the contralateral BAEPs well and detect the change in the waveform, you can observe more easily (Figs. 2.3 and 2.4).

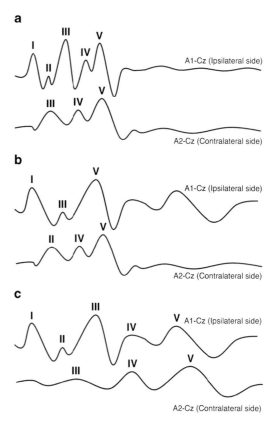

Fig. 2.3 During surgery, BAEPs should not be performed only at the surgical site. The BAEPs waveform is anatomically formed on both the ipsilateral and contralateral sides (**a**). Therefore, when a small change in the waveform occurs due to surgery, the ipsilateral waveform should be evaluated by comparing it with the contralateral side. (**b**) and (**c**) have the same ipsilateral side waveform. However, the waveform on the contralateral side is completely different. Therefore, it is good to measure and compare the waveform of the contralateral side to determine the ipsilateral side waveform correctly. BAEPs test with only the ipsilateral side waveform may overlook a serious condition

Very rarely, the waveform itself is not a pretty shape, so it is difficult to distinguish the waveform. Alternatively, there are cases where surgical manipulation of the surgical site affects the BAEPs waveform. Even in this case, if you observe the contralateral BAEPs well and detect the change in the waveform, you can observe more easily. In particular, despite the decrease or loss of the waveform, it may appear that the waveform of the BAEPs on the receiving site is small, so if you observe and compare the wave-

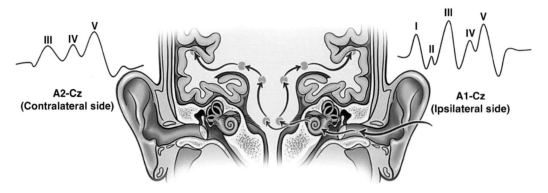

Fig. 2.4 The sound stimulus from one ear is separated into both sides and transmitted to both auditory cortex

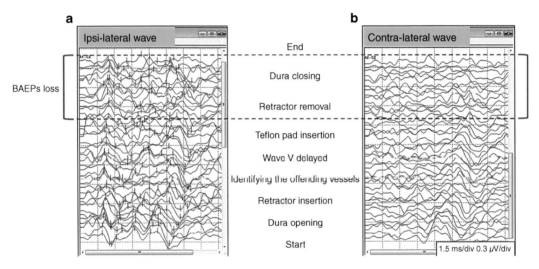

Fig. 2.5 For BAEPs wave loss, it is recommended to observe the ipsilateral wave (**a**) and the contralateral wave (**b**) at the same time

forms of the contralateral side, it can be very helpful to detect the change of the true BAEPs waveform (Fig. 2.5).

2.3 Optimal Test of Lateral Spread Response (LSR) by New Method

Electric stimulus flows from anode (+) to cathode (−) direction. And electrical stimulation occurs at the cathode (−). Therefore, the desired stimulation site should be located in the cathode (−) area.

The waveforms that occur according to the position of electrical stimulation to one nerve vary. When only the cathode is located on the nerve, the waveform is measured slightly smaller than the original (Fig. 2.6a). When only the anode is located on the nerve, the waveform is not formed or is measured very poorly (Fig. 2.6b). If neither anode nor cathode is located on the nerve, the waveform cannot be formed and the stimulation intensity must be increased to measure. However, if the intensity is very high and stimulated, other nerves in the vicinity may also be stimulated, causing an error in waveform measurement (Fig. 2.6c). When both anode and cathode are located on the nerve, the optimum waveform with the largest amplitude at the lowest intensity is measured (Fig. 2.6d).

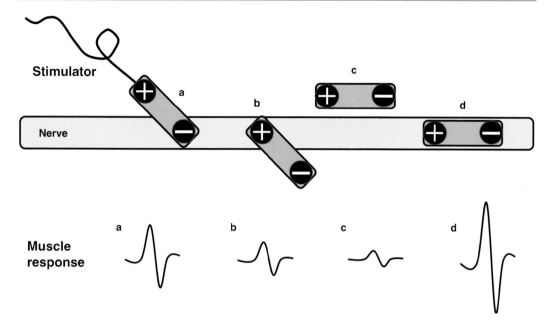

Fig. 2.6 Relationship with waveform according to nerve stimulation position

In most institutions facial nerve upper stimulate the temporal or zygomatic branch of the facial nerve about 3 cm lateral to the lateral margin of the orbit during LSR monitoring and facial nerve lower stimulate the buccal branch or mandibular branch of the facial nerve about 3 cm lateral to the oris muscle. The direction of stimulation with paired needles or surface electrodes is centripetal toward the brainstem with the cathode positioned proximally and a 0.2 to 0.3 ms stimulus with an intensity of 5 to 25 mA [14–18].

Then, let's look at the facial nerve branch selection method, stimulation direction, and stimulation intensity. What is the optimal test method for the LSR test that gives electrical stimulation to the facial nerve branch?

2.3.1   Optimal Choice of Stimulation Direction

In the preoperative test, when performing the LSR test while listening to the free-running EMG sound, patients with severe spasm may have difficulty discriminating by sound because the free-running EMG itself continuously produced an EMG sound too seriously. In addition, there were cases where the free-running EMG sound did not same from those where the LSR waveform was measured very well. So, we analyzed the electrical stimulation muscle response of the facial nerve branch where the electrical stimulation enters.

The conventional direction of electrical stimulation for LSR measurement is from the peripheral to the stem. In this way, the corresponding muscle response among frontalis, oculi, and oris, where electrodes are attached to the area where the electrical stimulation enters, is measured very small, making it difficult to determine whether the electrical stimulation is smoothly inserted into the nerve branch that you want to excite.

So, when the LSR stimulation direction was given from the stem to the peripheral direction, contrary to the previous one, the electrical stimulation muscle response was much larger and more clearly generated than before, so it was easy to grasp that the electrical stimulation was well transmitted to the corresponding nerve branch. The volume of the sound heard in the running EMG and the electrical stimulation muscle response were formed in proportion to satisfy both sound and waveform (Fig. 2.7).

a

b

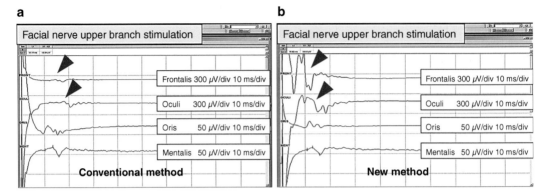

Fig. 2.7 The response measured in the frontalis and oculi muscles when the upper branch was stimulated by the conventional stimulation method was very small (**a**). The response measured in the frontalis and oculi muscles when the upper branch was stimulated by the new method stimulation was very large, making it easy to assess whether the upper branch was sufficiently excited (**b**)

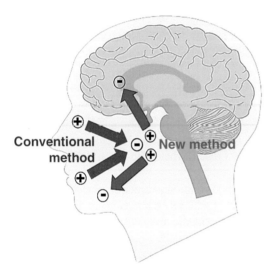

Fig. 2.8 The direction of stimulation in the conventional and the new methods. In the conventional method, electrodes are placed in the temporal or zygomatic branch of the facial nerve, about 3 cm lateral to the lateral margin of the orbit, and centripetal impulses are transmitted toward the brainstem with the cathode positioned proximally. In contrast, electrodes were inserted intradermally with the anode located proximally over the area just anterior to the mandibular fossa and the cathode located distally in the temporal branch of the facial nerve in the new method. The direction of stimulation was centrifugal outward from the brainstem

When the stimulation direction was stimulated from the stem to the peripheral direction, the LSR measurement was better when stimulating the temporal branch than the zygomatic branch when stimulating the facial nerve upper branch and when stimulating the facial nerve lower branch. LSR was measured better in the mandibular branch than in the buccal branch [19] (Fig. 2.8).

In particular, if the stimulation direction is measured in a way that stimulates the direction opposite to the conventional method, even during surgery, if the offending vessel is slightly separated from the facial nerve during surgery, the LSR immediately disappears. When the vessel is put back to its original position, the LSR is measured again. In this way, if the direction of the electrical stimulation is checked new method, the change in LSR is observed in a very sensitive way, so it is very advantageous in discriminating whether it is a true offending vessel.

2.3.2 Optimal Choice of Facial Nerve Branch

For optimal nerve action potentials, both the anode and cathode of the stimulator should be placed on the corresponding nerve. The same goes for the lateral spread response. When the facial nerve upper branch is sufficiently stimulated, the wave spread to the lower branch is well measured, and when the facial nerve lower branch is sufficiently stimulated, the wave spread to the upper branch is well measured.

When measuring LSR in the peripheral direction from the stem as a preoperative test, we selected a region where the waveform is formed in all ten times by stimulating ten times and the area measured at the lowest intensity that satisfies both criteria.

Several areas of the face were stimulated to find the optimal measurement area in the facial nerve branch of various patients, and while progressing in this manner, we found a common point in which LSR is well measured. It was found that when stimulating the area where LSR was best measured, the facial nerve branch where the electrical stimulation entered was the most excited.

In order to hear the sound of the free-running EMG, when the speaker is turned on and the test is performed, the muscle twitching sound is heard in the area where the electrical stimulation is applied. If the LSR response is well measured, the area where the facial nerve branch where the electrical stimulation is applied makes the loudest sound. This means that the LSR measurement is best when the facial nerve branch that has received electrical stimulation stimulates the place where it excites the most, and it means that both the anode and the cathode of the stimulator are well located on the corresponding nerve (Fig. 2.6).

When performing the LSR test from the stem to the peripheral direction before surgery preoperative test, it is recommended to turn on the speaker and find the place where the free-running EMG sound is the loudest.

2.3.3   Optimal Choice of Stimulation Intensity

When the depth of anesthesia is very smooth, the LSR can be measured even at 2 mA when the stimulation duration is 0.2 ms. In other words, it is often measured at very low intensity. If the LSR test is performed by increasing the intensity, the LSR can be measured even at 30 mA or higher, but the shape is slightly different from the LSR shape measured at low intensity.

However, the LSR measured when stimulating with a high intensity of 30 mA or more is not lost even after decompression and is often measured as it is. In this case, I think that it is not an LSR but a waveform that looks similar to an arti-

ficially generated LSR because all of the surrounding nerve branches are stimulated by strong electrical stimulation.

We know that, as mentioned in many papers on the branch of the facial nerve, the fine strands of the facial nerve are often connected to different facial nerves and the shape of the branch varies [20] (Fig. 2.9).

Therefore, it is recommended to check the LSR test by measuring the intensity section where the waveform is measured and finding the threshold that is the lowest intensity measured first. This is because the sensitivity of the LSR test can be made the highest when performing this test.

The purpose of the LSR test is to evaluate whether the operation was successful. If LSR is lost long after Teflon intervention, it is inappropriate to assess whether the operation went well. It is recommended to perform an LSR test with threshold intensity as the effect of the surgical operation can be directly reflected in the LSR to facilitate the operation.

If the abovementioned stimulation direction, facial nerve branch selection method, and the new method of test with stimulation intensity threshold are attempted, the efficiency of the LSR test will be enhanced, thereby helping a safer and more complete surgery [19].

To summarize the new method, contrary to the conventional method, when stimulation of the facial nerve upper branch is performed, electrical stimulation is applied to the frontalis and oculi muscles to find and examine the place where the facial nerve upper branch is sufficiently excited.

In order to use the same area during surgery as the area where LSR is well measured by performing a preoperative test, we fix the temporomandibular joint area with the anode electrode and move the cathode electrode area in a fan shape to ensure that LSR is well measured to find the site and examine it.

Although not described in the paper, facial nerve lower branch stimulation is located by fixing the molar part with the anode electrode and moving the cathode electrode part in a fan shape to find and examine the optimal part where LSR is well measured. Because parotid impairs facial nerve lower branch stimulation, the LSR response is better

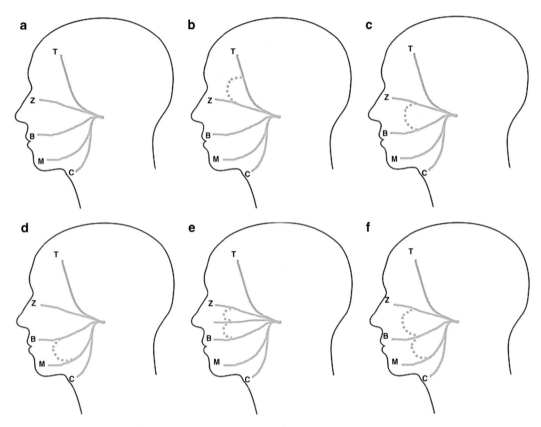

Fig. 2.9 Illustration of branching pattern of the facial nerve six categories. T, temporal branch; Z, zygomatic branch; B, buccal branch; M, mandibular branch; and C, cervical branch. The phenomenon in which the facial nerves are finely connected to each other is divided into six major categories. (**a**) is the basic shape of the branches of the facial nerve, (**b**) is a shape in which temporal branch and zygomatic branch are finely connected to each other, (**c**) is the shape that the zygomatic branch and the buccal branch are finely connected to each other, (**d**) is a shape in which the buccal branch and mandibular branch are finely connected to each other, (**e**) is the shape that the buccal branch is very developed and is finely connected to the zygomatic branch, (**f**) is a shape in which zygomatic branch, buccal branch, and mandibular branch are finely connected to each other

measured when stimulating the mandibular branch than when the buccal branch is stimulated [21].

2.4   The Free-Running EMG Waveform Continues to Fluctuate. Why Is This?

Optimal Electrode Insertion Method for Facial Nerve EMG Measurement

The subdermal needle electrode should be inserted into the distal area of the facial nerve and fixed so that it cannot be removed or moved (Fig. 2.10). If it falls out slightly, there is a lot of mixing of electrical artifacts in the surrounding area (Fig. 2.11), and the effect of the disinfectant used to clean the surgical site can be more severe (Figs. 2.12 and 2.13). When the electrode is completely removed, the impedance measurement value is displayed as more than 25 kΩ, so it can be distinguished. However, the electrode that is only slightly removed to the middle of the needle cannot be distinguished because the impedance measurement value is less than 2.5 kΩ. Therefore, it is necessary to insert the electrode well, taking care not to fall out slightly.

2.4.1   Correct Electrode Insertion Method

For the frontalis muscle, an electrode is inserted in the area raised above the orbital outermost ear or an average of 4 cm above the tip of the eyebrow, and the orbicularis oculi is inserted in the upper part of the orbit or the upper eyebrow. Orbicularis oris is difficult to insert under the lip due to the intubation tube, so it is inserted into the upper lip. Since the thickness of the upper part of the lip is thin, care should be taken not to let the electrode pass through the flesh and enter the mouth. When the electrode enters the mouth, it may bleed, or the free-running EMG waveform is continuously shaken due to saliva. Mentalis position must be placed between the upper and lower lip by touching the jawbone. Since the intubation tube pushes the lower lip a lot, the mentalis area is difficult to see smoothly. Therefore, it is often the case that the electrode is installed below the original mentalis muscle. In particular, people who are overweight make the mistake of inserting electrodes on the neck, not mentalis, because the shape of the jaw shown is mixed with the neck. Mentalis site is the LSR site that must be observed most carefully when stimulation of the upper branch of the facial nerve, so it must be well inserted (Fig. 2.10).

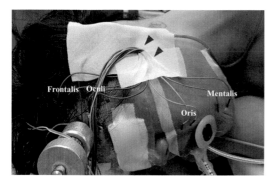

Fig. 2.10. Subdermal needle electrode insertion of facial nerve EMG

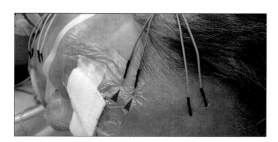

Fig. 2.11 Illustration of the orbicularis oculi electrode slightly missing

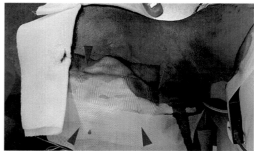

Fig. 2.12 Facial nerve EMG. Completely tape the attached part so that it does not come off or get wet with the disinfectant solution

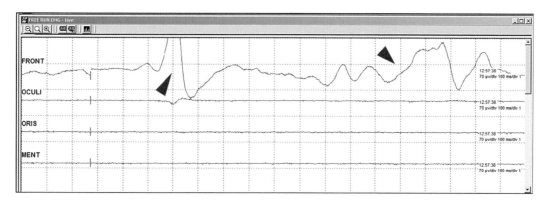

Fig. 2.13 A figure in which a disinfectant enters a slightly missing frontalis electrode and affects the waveform

The patient was well-observed in the LSR test before surgery of preoperative test. If there is a case where the LSR waveform is not observed at all in mentalis even when the facial nerve upper branch stimulation is performed while the depth of anesthesia is smooth during the surgery, it may be because the position of the electrode inserted into the mentalis is inappropriate. In this case, if you slightly change the electrode position of mentalis, the LSR waveform may suddenly be well measured.

References

1. Joo BE, Park SK, Cho KR, Kong DS, Seo DW, Park K. Real-time intraoperative monitoring of brainstem auditory evoked potentials during microvascular decompression for hemifacial spasm. J Neurosurg. 2016;125:1061–1067. https://doi.org/10.3171/2015.10.JNS151224. Epub 2016 Jan 29.
2. Raudzens PA, Shetter AG. Intraoperative monitoring of brain-stem auditory evoked potentials. J Neurosurg. 1982 Sep;57(3):341–8. https://doi.org/10.3171/jns.1982.57.3.0341.
3. Grundy BL, Jannetta PJ, Procopio PT, Lina A, Boston JR, Doyle E. Intraoperative monitoring of brain-stem auditory evoked potentials. J Neurosurg. 1982 Nov;57(5):674–81. https://doi.org/10.3171/jns.1982.57.5.0674.
4. Watanabe E, Schramm J, Strauss C, Fahlbusch R. Neurophysiologic monitor-ing in posterior fossa surgery: part II-BAEP-waves I and V and preservation of hearing. Acta Neurochir. 1989;98(3–4):118–28. https://doi.org/10.1007/BF01407337.
5. Polo G, Fischer C, Sindou MP, Marneffe V. Brainstem auditory evoked potential monitoring during microvascular decompression for hemifacial spasm: intraoperative brainstem auditory evoked potential changes and warning values to prevent hearing loss—prospective study in a consecutive series of 84 patients. Neurosurgery. 2004 Jan;54(1):97–104. https://doi.org/10.1227/01.neu.0000097268.90620.07; discussion 104–6.
6. Polo G, Fische C. Intraoperative monitoring of brainstem auditory evoked potentials during microvascular decompression of cranial nerves in cerebellopontine angle. Neurochirurgie. 2009 Apr;55(2):152–157. https://doi.org/10.1016/j.neuchi.2009.01.005. Epub 2009 Mar 18.
7. Legatt AD. Mechanisms of intraoperative brainstem auditory evoked potential changes. J Clin Neurophysiol. 2002 Oct;19(5):396–408. https://doi.org/10.1097/00004691-200210000-00003.
8. Jo KW, Kim JW, Kong DS, Hong SH, Park K. The patterns and risk factors of hearing loss following micro-vascular decompression for hemifacial spasm. Acta Neurochir. 2011 May;153(5):1023–1030. https://doi.org/10.1007/s00701-010-0935-8. Epub 2011 Jan 15.
9. Jung NY, Lee SW, Park CK, Chang WS, Jung HH, Chang JW. Hearing outcome following microvascular decompression for hemifacial spasm: series of 1434 cases. World Neurosurg. 2017 Dec;108:566–571. https://doi.org/10.1016/j.wneu.2017.09.053. Epub 2017 Sep 18.
10. Park SK, Joo BE, Lee S, Lee, JA, Hwang JH, Kong DS, Seo DW, Park K, Lee HT. The critical warning sign of real-time brainstem auditory evoked potentials during microvascular decompression for hemifacial spasm. Clin Neurophysiol. 2018 May;129(5):1097–1102. https://doi.org/10.1016/j.clinph.2017.12.032. Epub 2018 Jan 4.
11. Martin WH, Stecker MM. ASNM position statement: intraoperative monitoring of auditory evoked potentials. J Clin Monit Comput. 2008 Feb;22(1):75–85. https://doi.org/10.1007/s10877-007-9108-6.
12. Society AE. Guideline eleven: guidelines for intraoperative monitoring of sensory evoked potentials. J Clin Neurophysiol. 1994 Jan;11(1):77–87.
13. Møller AR, Jannetta PJ. Neural generators of auditory evoked potentials. In: Jacobson JT, editor. The auditory brainstem response. SanDiego: College-Hill Press; 1985. p. 13–31.
14. Møller AR, Jannetta PJ. Monitoring facial EMG responses during microvascular decompression operations for hemifacial spasm. J Neurosurg. 1987 May;66(5):681–5. https://doi.org/10.3171/jns.1987.66.5.0681.
15. Wilkinson MF, Kaufmann AM. Monitoring of facial muscle motor evoked potentials during microvascular decompression for hemifacial spasm: evidence of changes in motor neuron excitability. J Neurosurg. 2005 Jul;103(1):64–9. https://doi.org/10.3171/jns.2005.103.1.0064.
16. Damaty AE, Rosenstengel C, Matthes M, Baldauf J, Schroeder HWS. The value of lateral spread response monitoring in predicting the clinical outcome after microvascular decompression in hemifacial spasm: a prospective study on 100 patients. Neurosurg Rev. 2016;39:455–466. https://doi.org/10.1007/s10143-016-0708-9. Epub 2016 Apr 6.
17. Lee SH, Park BJ, Shin HS, Park CK, Rhee BA, Lim YJ. Prognostic ability of intraoperative electromyographic monitoring during microvascular decompression for hemifacial spasm to predict lateral spread response outcome. J Neurosurg. 2017 Feb;126(2):391–396. https://doi.org/10.3171/2016.1.JNS151782. Epub 2016 Apr 22.
18. von Eckardstein K, Harper C, Castner M, Link M. The significance of intraoperative electromyographic "lateral spread" in predicting outcome of microvascular decompression for hemifacial spasm. J Neurol Surg B Skull Base. 2014 Jun;75(3):198–203. https://doi.org/10.1055/s-0034-1368145. Epub 2014 Mar 12.
19. Lee S, Park SK, Lee JA, Joo BE, Kong DS, Seo DW, Park K. A new method for monitoring abnormal

muscle response in hemifacial spasm: A prospective study. Clin Neurophysiol. 2018 Jul;129(7):1490–1495. https://doi.org/10.1016/j.clinph.2018.03.006. Epub 2018 Mar 27.

20. Katz AD, Catalano P. The clinical significance of the various anastomotic branches of the facial nerve. report of 100 patients. Arch Otolaryngol Head Neck Surg. 1987 Sep;113(9):959–62. https://doi.org/10.1001/archotol.1987.01860090057019.

21. Gataa IS, Faris BJM. Patterns and surgical significance of facial nerve branching within the parotid gland in 43 cases. Oral Maxillofac Surg. 2016 Jun;20(2):161–165. https://doi.org/10.1007/s10006-015-0543-0. Epub 2016 Jan 11.

Cases of Brainstem Auditory Evoked Potentials

3.1 What Is the Difference Between the Case Where the Latency Is Continuously Delayed, the Amplitude Decreases Gradually, and Then the BAEP Loss or Suddenly BAEP Loss Occurs? And Which One Is More Dangerous?

What is the continuously gradually BAEPs change pattern and the suddenly occurs pattern

It is rare that there is no change in the BAEP waveform at all during surgery. In most surgeries, the change in waveform is always observed subtly. Waveform change can be divided into a case where it changes rapidly and a case where it changes slowly, and it can be classified into three temporal concepts.

Phase I: Looking at the case where the surgery proceeds stably, there is no change in the wave V amplitude, and only the wave V latency is <1 ms, and little changes are observed in most surgery. At all times, the change in latency gradually progresses continuously for several minutes to several tens of minutes, and after the main procedure is finished, the original waveform gradually recovers.

Phase II: During the main procedure, when affected by the brain retractor or manipulation, the wave V latency, which was slowly extended very little by little, is observed to extend more than 1 ms. However, the wave V amplitude decreases by more than 50% of the wave V amplitude very quickly within 10 s, unlike the latency, which is gradually observed.

Phase III: In the main procedure, when the offending site is difficult to see or the decompression position is the facial nerve ventral side, if excessive use of the brain retractor causes a lot of influence on the cochlear nerve, BAEP wave V loss occurs very quickly and suddenly.

Below, we divided the phase by phase and compared the waveform change and the postoperative hearing.

3.1.1 Phase I Only Slowly and Continuously Observed and Then Recovered

The BAEP change of the extent that the wave V latency extension of <1 ms and the amplitude decrease to <50% accounts for more than 50% of all MVD patients, and all postoperative hearing is normal (Fig. 3.1).

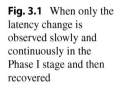

Fig. 3.1 When only the latency change is observed slowly and continuously in the Phase I stage and then recovered

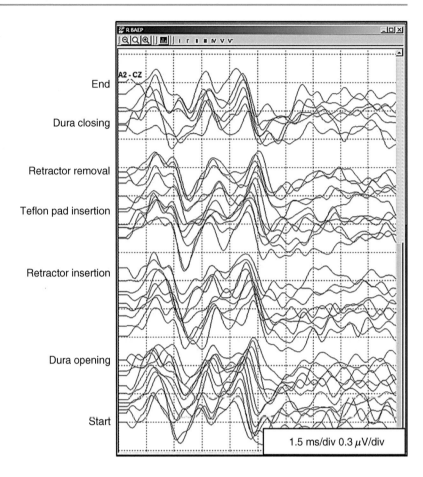

3.1.2 Phase II Suddenly Observed and Recovered After Phase I

After dura open, the waveform was well-observed without any change in wave V amplitude during the main procedure. During the Teflon-felt insertion process, the amplitude suddenly decreased by more than 50%, and the latency was extended by more than 1 ms and then gradually recovered. Most patients have normal hearing after surgery. However, very occasionally, low-frequency hearing decreased by 10 dB after surgery (0.2% in our experience) (Fig. 3.2).

3.1.3 If Phase III Is Suddenly Observed While Leading to Phase II After Phase I

In the process of approach after dura open, only latency was continuously observed without change in wave V amplitude, and the shape of the waveform became poor, and the amplitude of the waveform decreased by 50% and abrupt wave loss. After the operation, the patient developed deafness (Fig. 3.3).

3.1.4 If Phase I Is Observed Continuously Slowly and Suddenly Phase III Is Observed

In the process of approach after dura open, only latency was gradually extended over 2 ms without change in wave V amplitude. During the insertion of the Teflon-felt, a sudden decrease of more than 80% in amplitude was observed, and the waveform was immediately lost. After the main procedure, the retractor was removed, and the waveform was waiting for recovery, but the waveform was not recovered. After the operation, the patient developed deafness (Fig. 3.4).

Fig. 3.2 When Phase II is suddenly observed and recovered after Phase I

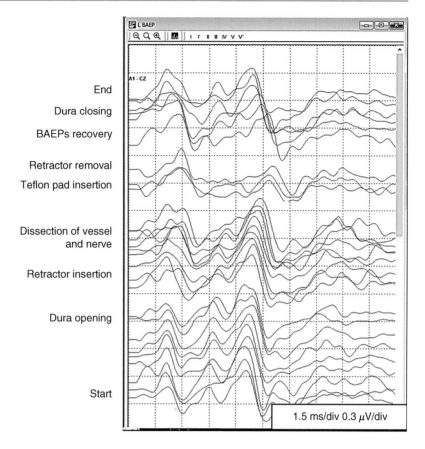

End

Dura closing

BAEPs recovery

Retractor removal
Teflon pad insertion

Dissection of vessel and nerve

Retractor insertion

Dura opening

Start

1.5 ms/div 0.3 μV/div

3.1.5   Phase II Observed Without Phase I and Suddenly Phase III Observed

After opening the dura, the waveform was well-observed without any change in wave V amplitude during the main procedure, but the shape of the waveform suddenly became unstable and then rapidly disappeared (Fig. 3.5).

We waited for the waveform to recover until the end of the operation, but the waveform did not recover. After the operation, the patient developed deafness.

3.1.6   When Phase III Is Observed Suddenly Without Phase I

After opening the dura, the waveform was well-observed without any change in wave V amplitude during the main procedure, but the shape of

the waveform suddenly became unstable and then rapidly disappeared. We waited for the waveform to recover until the end of the operation, but the waveform did not recover. After the operation, the patient developed deafness (Fig. 3.6).

3.1.7   Without Phase I, II, and III and When the Waveform Suddenly Becomes Unstable and Recovers

During the main procedure, the waveform was well-observed without any change in wave V amplitude. After closing the dura, the shape of the waveform suddenly jumped very irregularly for a while, and then the waveform was measured normally before the operation was completed. High-frequency HL occurred after surgery. We believe that the BAEP waveform became irregu-

Fig. 3.3 Phase III is
observed suddenly after
Phase I followed by
Phase II

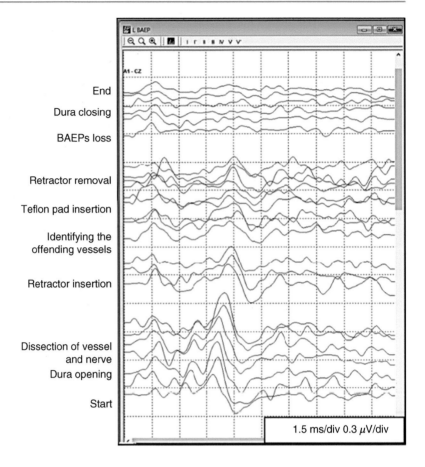

Fig. 3.4 When Phase I
is observed slowly and
then suddenly Phase III
is observed

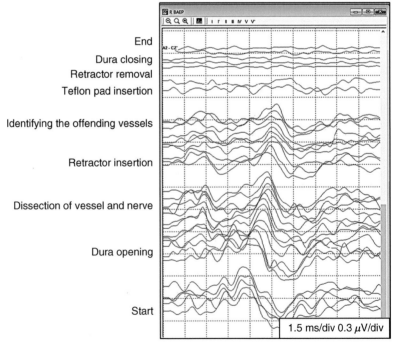

Fig. 3.5 Without Phase I, Phase II is observed, and then Phase III is suddenly observed

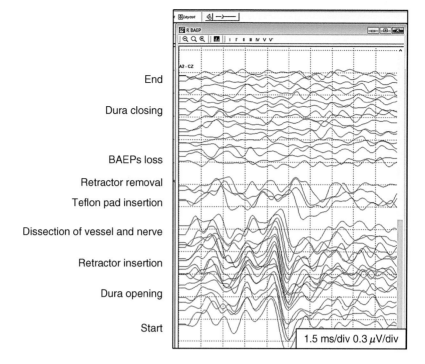

Fig. 3.6 Abrupt Phase III observation without Phase I

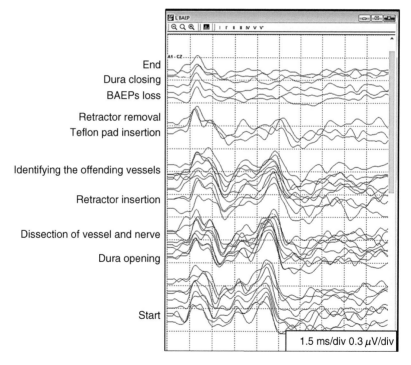

lar due to temporary vasospasm at the end of the operation due to this cause, and for this reason, high-frequency HL occurred after the operation (Fig. 3.7).

3.1.7.1 Conclusion

In the case of Phase I, where only the prolongation of wave V latency is observed very slowly and continuously, it accounts for more than half

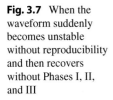

Fig. 3.7 When the waveform suddenly becomes unstable without reproducibility and then recovers without Phases I, II, and III

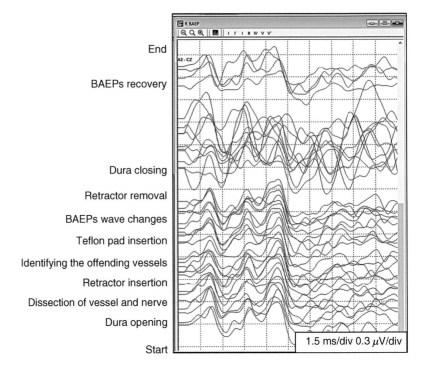

of all surgeries, and this phenomenon can be observed even with dura open only. In general, BAEP wave change can be divided into traumatic damage and vascular circulation damage.

Waveform changes due to traumatic mechanical damage are observed in all phases, Phase I, II, and III, and can be classified into four stages, mild, moderate, severe, and critical damage according to the degree of direct damage to the cochlear nerve.

- Mild damage i.s a Phase I stage, showing only wave V latency delayed. A slight decrease in amplitude is observed, but it recovers immediately to the original waveform shape.
- Moderate damage is Phase II in which Phase I is further advanced, and it is observed from the wave V latency delayed state to an additional 50% decrease in wave V amplitude. The reason for presenting the criterion of wave V amplitude 50% in Phase II is that when the wave V amplitude decreases by 50%, the wave V amplitude recovers easily if the effect caused by the main procedure is removed. In other words, when the wave V amplitude is reduced by 50% or more, if left as it is, the

waveform may further decrease or the waveform may be lost. And in this state, even if any effort is made to recover the waveform, it is often not possible to recover to a normal waveform again, and it takes a very long time to recover. So, we consider the criterion of wave V amplitude 50% as the amplitude reversible point (Fig. 3.8).

- Severe damage can be classified into several types.
- Severe damage-1: Wave V latency delayed is more than 2 ms, and wave V amplitude is reduced by more than 80%. When the wave V latency delayed is more than 2 ms, there are many cases where the wave V amplitude suddenly decreases. Therefore, be very careful and observe the waveform change. An 80% reduction in wave V amplitude means a state in which wave V amplitude measurement is barely possible. In other words, it means the state of the smallest amplitude can be said to have a waveform, and if the main procedure continues when such a waveform is observed, most waveforms are lost.
- Severe damage-2: Phase II suddenly occurs without going through Phase I. If focal damage occurs severely, the amplitude suddenly

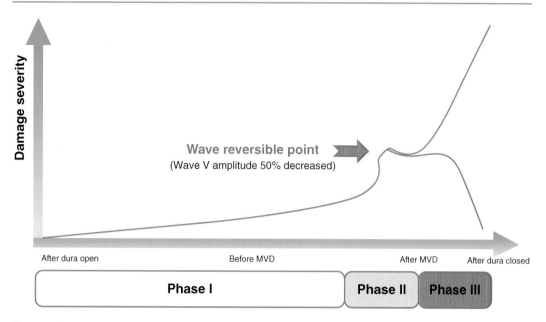

Fig. 3.8 Only wave V latency delayed ≤1 ms (Phase I), wave V latency delayed ≥1 ms with wave V amplitude 50% decreased (Phase II), wave V loss (Phase III)

decreases without changing the latency of wave V. We often experienced a case where the wave V amplitude suddenly decreased by more than 50%, and when this occurred, the waveform could not recover well or lead to wave V amplitude loss.

- Severe damage-3: It is a change in the waveform due to vascular circulation damage. Without Phase I or II, the reproducibility of the waveform suddenly disappears. In other words, it refers to the state of the waveform that swells like dancing without observing the I, III, and V waveforms of the BAEP wave. In this case, the inspectors may think that the electrode is missing or caused by external artifacts, so they may be left unattended and continued. If there is a change in the morphology of the waveform of BAEPs, it is because a disorder occurs in the vascular circulation. In this case, a vasodilator such as papaverin should be administered to smooth the vascular circulation flow of the surrounding blood vessels. Otherwise, if left unattended, a loss of total wave that is not observed will be observed, and after the operation, patients will witness a deaf patient complaining of a general disorder of the vestibular system.

- Critical damage is a phenomenon in which both traumatic mechanical damage and vascular circulation damage occur, and BAEP loss occurs. Even if any waveform change occurs during surgery, the patient's hearing is fine as long as the waveform is observed at the end of the surgery. However, almost all patients become deaf after surgery when the waveform is lost, the operation is not recovered, and the operation is terminated.

Each phase has its own characteristic; Phase I is that the wave V latency is extended slowly and continuously for several minutes to several tens of minutes. There was no change in hearing after surgery due to this Phase I effect. We think this slow change is due to a very weak effect. However, contrary to this, in Phase II, the wave V amplitude suddenly decreases by 50% within 10 s. In the case of Phase III, it is a very rare phenomenon to pass through Phase I and then to Phase II and to Phase III, and most of the observations of Phase III are observed abruptly. In other words, in BAEP wave, latency corresponds to slow change, and amplitude corresponds to fast change. Therefore, to classify the importance of waveform change in terms of time, it can be said that the observation of the amplitude corresponding to the fast change is more important.

In addition, it is a much more dangerous situation when there is no change in waveform, and then suddenly a change in latency or amplitude is observed. In most cases when a change in wave V latency of a waveform is observed, then a decrease in wave V amplitude is observed sequentially. Even when analyzing the state in which the waveform changes and the waveform recovers after the main procedure is finished, when the waveform suddenly changes, it takes much longer to recover, or the recovery is not complete, and the surgery is often terminated. It is similar to the case where the waveform is lost. In the case where both wave V latency and wave V amplitude changes are observed and lead to disappearance, the waveform is often recovered gradually after the main procedure is finished. However, if there is no change in any waveform and then suddenly disappears, it is considered dangerous because most of the surgery is terminated without recovery, and there are more HL after surgery.

Taking all of these situations together, it is dangerous to change the waveform suddenly and abruptly, and even if the waveform is lost, it is much more dangerous to lose it suddenly.

The BAEP test should be conducted so that it is repeated continuously and rapidly so that it will be easy to detect sudden changes in a short time (Table 3.1).

Table 3.1 Explain the relationship between phase and nerve damage degree, which is a temporal classification, as a change in waveform

	Damage degree	Latency change		Amplitude change
Phase I	Mild	≤1 ms		≤50%
Phase II	Moderate	≥1 ms		≥50%
	Severe	1	≥2 ms	≥80%
		2	No change	≥50% (abrupt change)
		3	No reproducibility	
Phase III	Critical	1	Loss—traumatic mechanical damage	
		2	Loss—vascular circulation damage	

3.2 What Is More Important About the Latency and Amplitude of Wave V for BAEPs Change?

New warning criteria

We are well aware that changes in the BAEP waveform during surgery are very diverse. And I am very curious about how these waveform changes are related to the patient's hearing after surgery.

Existing well-known warning criteria are the 1 ms extension of wave V latency, 50% reduction in amplitude, and loss of wave V [1, 2].

We performed the test in the real-time BAEP method [3], and because of that, we were able to detect the waveform change during surgery very quickly. In the last 2 years, 606 patients who had undergone MVD surgery after visiting hemifacial spasm were observed for changes in BAEP waveforms during surgery, and they could be divided into six groups as follows (Table 3.2).

Group 1.   Wave V latency prolongation of <1 ms and amplitude reduction of <50%, 346 patients, 57.1% of the total, except that one patient had low-frequency HL. All other patients had the same normal postoperative hearing.

Group 2.   Wave V latency prolonged for more than 2 ms, and amplitude decreased by <50%, 38 patients, 6.3% of the total, and no change in hearing after surgery.

Group 3.   When only the wave V amplitude was reduced by 50% or more, 15

Table 3.2 BAEP groups of change patterns

Group	Latency	Amplitude
1	≤1 ms	≤50%
2	≥2 ms	≤50%
3	≤1 ms	≥50%
4	≥2 ms	≥50%
5	Permanent loss	
6	Transient loss	

BAEP wave V standard

Table 3.3 Distribution of waveform changes

	0 ms	1 ms	1.5 ms	2 ms	2.5 ms	3 ms
0%	346	83	27	32	6	0
50%	17	2	3	34	0	2
80%	3	2	6	10	3	2
Loss	22 (4)	2	1	3 (1)	0	0

The number in parentheses is deaf

sient loss were 3.8% of the total, and there were no patients with total deafness after surgery, and high-frequency hearing loss (10 dB reduction) was observed in 4 patients (Table 3.3).

patients had 2.5% of the total, and all postoperative hearing was normal.

Group 4.   When the latency was prolonged by 2 ms and the amplitude was reduced by more than 50%, 36 patients (5.9%) and 1 postoperative deafness occurred.

Group 5.   When the amplitude loss occurred and did not recover, it was 0.83% of the total in five patients, and deafness occurred after the operation.

Group 6.   When amplitude loss occurred and recovered, 23 patients with tran-

3.2.1   (Group 1) If Not Applicable to Warning Criteria

However, in one patient, low-frequency hearing loss (10 dB reduction) was observed after surgery (Fig. 3.9).

3.2.2   (Group 2) In Case Only the Status of Warning Criteria Has Been Delayed by 2 ms (Fig. 3.10)

Fig. 3.9 Wave V latency was prolonged by <1 ms and amplitude decreased to <50%, and then 346 patients recovered to normal, and 57.1% of the total showed no change in hearing after surgery

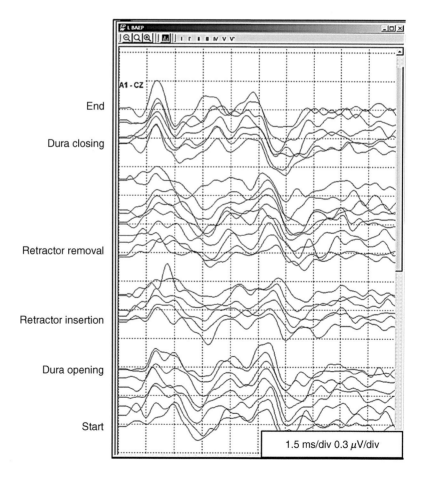

Fig. 3.10 There were 38 patients who recovered to normal after having extended wave V latency of 2 ms or more and decreased amplitude by <50%. There was no change in hearing after surgery (6.3%)

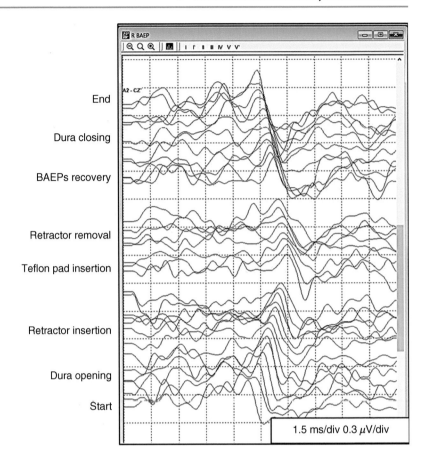

3.2.3 (Group 3) In the Case Where the Amplitude Was Reduced by More Than 50% (Fig. 3.11)

3.2.4 (Group 4) In the Case of Delayed Latency 2 ms and Reduced Amplitude by More Than 50%

In one deaf patient, waveform change was observed during surgery and recovered normally. However, as the postoperative vertigo was severe and accompanied by deafness symptoms, it is estimated that vascular circulation disorder occurred in the vestibule–cochlear system after the surgery was completed (Fig. 3.12).

3.2.5 (Group 5) In the Case Where Amplitude Loss Occurs and Is Not Recovered (Fig. 3.13)

3.2.6 (Group 6) In the Case Where Amplitude Loss Occurs and Is Recovered (Fig. 3.14)

3.2.6.1 Conclusion

In real-time BAEP tests, it is observed that the latency of wave V is very slow and continuously delayed to <1 ms in most patients.

Rarely, it is also observed that the latency of wave V is delayed more than 3 ms (Fig. 3.15). These changes in latency gradually recovered to the normal waveform after the main procedure

Fig. 3.11 There were 15 patients who had a wave V latency prolongation of 1 ms or less and a waveform change that returned to normal after a decrease of more than 50% in amplitude (2.5%), and all postoperative hearing was normal

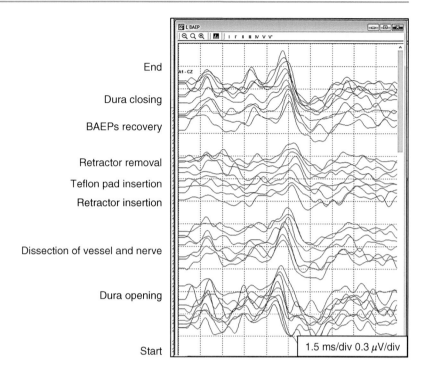

Fig. 3.12 Wave V latency of 2 ms or more and amplitude change of 50% or more were observed at the same time, and then the number of patients recovered was 36, 5.9% of the total, and 1 postoperative deafness occurred

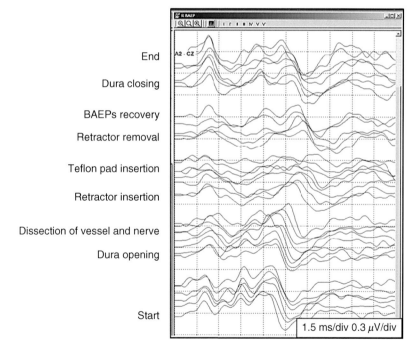

Fig. 3.13 The number of patients who could not recover due to wave V amplitude loss and completed the operation was 0.83% of the total and all the patient deaf occurred after the operation

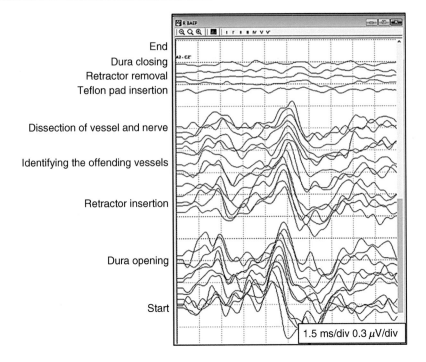

Fig. 3.14 The number of transient loss patients who recovered from the occurrence of wave V amplitude loss was 23 patients, 3.8% of the total. Postoperative high-frequency hearing loss (10 dB reduction) was observed in 4 patients after surgery, and the remaining patients without total deaf patients. All had normal hearing

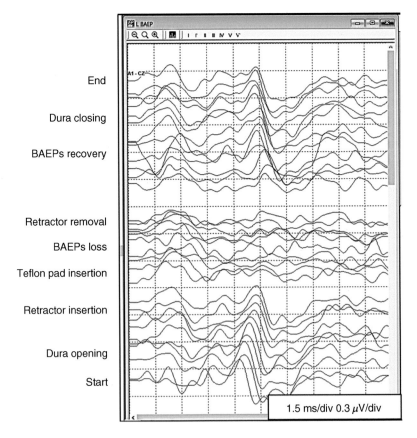

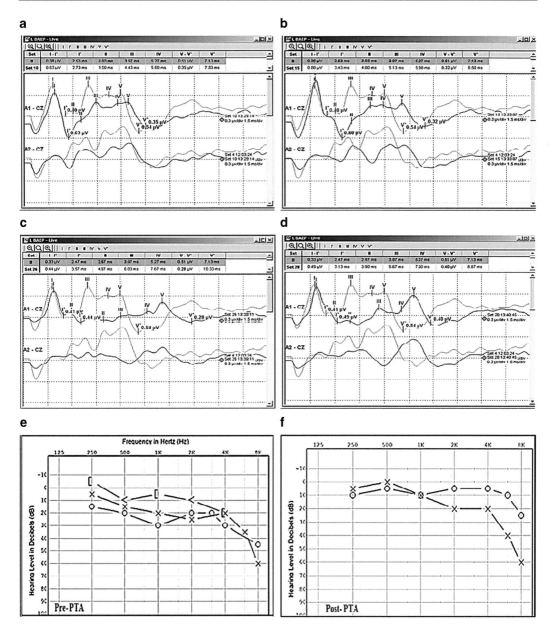

Fig. 3.15 A representative case showing only latency prolongation (≥1 ms) without a significant change in amplitude (the latency of wave V was delayed by 3.20 ms from 7.13 to 10.33 ms with a minimal decrease in the amplitude). The patient in this example did not experience postoperative hearing loss. (The average pre-PTA threshold was 22.5 dB, and the average post-PTA threshold was 6.25 dB). (**a–d**) The INM of BAEP during MVD surgery (*green line* = baseline of wave V; *black line* = wave V showing maximal prolongation in latency), (**e**) pre operative pure tone audiometry (**f**) pure tone audiometry of the patients obtained prior to surgery and 7 days postoperatively

was completed, and all of them were normal when examining the hearing after surgery.

In contrast, the amplitude of wave V was frequently observed to change more than 50% abruptly within a short time of about 10 s. In other words, it will be difficult to observe the amplitude that rapidly decreases from about 10 s in the conventional method that takes about 100 s to averaging the BAEP test 1000 times and then performing the test at 10 Hz. However, little by little, the latency, which is continuously delayed, can be observed as a waveform no matter what inspection method is performed.

Deafness occurred in 1 of 36 patients who recovered to normal after prolonging the latency by 2 ms and decreasing the amplitude by more than 50%. All five patients with permanent loss with wave V loss developed deafness after surgery. High-frequency hearing loss (10 dB reduction) was observed in 4 out of 23 transient loss patients whose wave V loss became temporary and recovered. From this point of view, it is difficult to define which is more important between the latency and amplitude of BAEP wave V. However, it is thought that it is more important to observe the amplitude at which the change occurs rapidly within 10 s rather than the latency at which the change is gradually observed. The change in latency always occurs first, followed by the change in amplitude over time. In particular, we can often observe a sudden decrease in amplitude when the latency is extended by more than 2 ms. In particular, all permanent wave V loss deafness occurred. Therefore, latency and amplitude are considered to be closely related, and the following warning criteria are proposed (Fig. 3.16) [4].

3.3   Can a Prewarning Sign from a BAEP Test Predict a Significant Change in the Waveform in Advance?

Prewarning sign in BAEP wave changes

The criterion for measuring the change of BAEP waveform is judged as the main criterion for the latency and amplitude change of wave V [5]. Looking at the case where the wave V latency is extended by more than 1 ms and then recovers, in some cases it recovers almost similar to the base data, and in some cases, the operation is finished with a delayed latency without recovering close to the base data. There are cases where the surgery is terminated with a body with a decreased amplitude. It is thought that the cochlear nerve is not seriously damaged unless BAEPs are lost. Let's look at why there is a difference in the resilience of the waveform.

Wave V is the waveform recorded in the inferior colliculus of the midbrain after passing through several synapses. In addition, since all surgeries during MVD for HFS are performed at

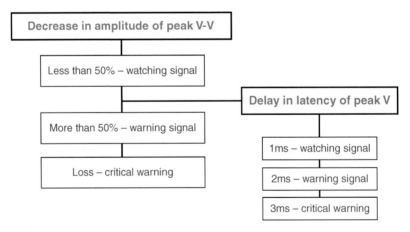

Fig. 3.16 Correlation of amplitude and latency in warning criteria. Warning criteria applied when using real-time BAEP. The relationship between latency and amplitude is presented separately based on wave V. In real-time BAEP tests, latency changes were always observed first, followed by amplitude changes. In addition, latency change was observed slowly and continuously, and amplitude changes suddenly decreased by more than 50% within 10 s

the muscle exit (REZ) of the facial nerve, damage to the auditory pathway during MVD will first cause a change in BAEP wave I or wave III. Therefore, analyzing changes to wave I or III before significant changes to wave V occur will be useful to more quickly identify the risk of HL after surgery.

In particular, cerebellar retraction to access the cerebellopontine angle is the most common mechanism of postoperative HL during MVD [6–8]. When performing MVD retraction, two different patterns are observed in BAEP depending on the direction in which CN VIII is pulled. When CN VIII is pulled to the brainstem, the change of BAEP occurs in wave I, and when CN VIII is pulled to the brainstem, the change of BAEP occurs in wave III, not wave I (Fig. 3.17).

When examining the patients whose BAEP wave V latency was extended by more than 1 ms, they were classified into two groups (Fig. 3.18).

Group I is the group that changed the wave V latency due to the change in the wave I latency delayed and the waves I–V inter-peak latency slightly prolonged.

Group II is the wave I latency did not change as it is, and the waves I–III inter-peak latency prolonged a lot.

In order to define the prewarning value for the change in wave I or wave III, the previous BAEP

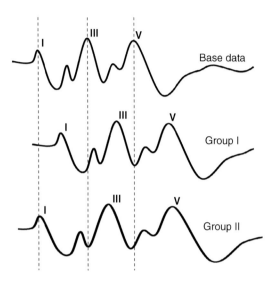

Fig. 3.17 When the vestibulocochlear nerve is ground in the brainstem direction, it is delayed from wave I (Gr I), and when the brainstem itself is ground, it is delayed from wave III (Gr II)

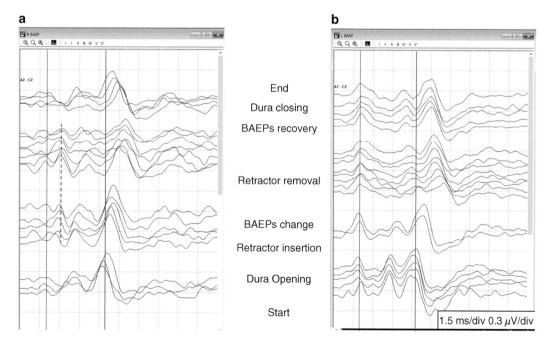

Fig. 3.18 Group I extends from wave I and recovers well from wave V at the end of surgery (**a**), group II extends from wave III, and at the end of surgery, wave V does not recover well (**b**)

Table 3.4 BAEPs by group transient loss, permanent loss, and hearing loss

	Group I		Group II	
n (241)	81		160	
Wave V loss	Transient loss	Permanent loss	Transient loss	Permanent loss
	24 (29.6%)	1 (1.2%)	32 (20.0%)	10 (6.3%)
Hearing loss	0	0	2 (1.2%)	3 (1.9%)

was analyzed before the significant change in wave V occurred in patients with a significant change in wave V during MVD, and the evaluation criterion was the change in wave V latency. If the wave V latency difference between the base data and the closing data was recovered within 0.5 ms, it was evaluated that it recovered well.

There are differences between the two groups due to changes in BAEP. In BAEP's maximal change analysis, there were 81 people in group I who showed change from wave I and 160 people in group II who showed change from wave III. However, the incidence of wave V loss was 26 (31.7%) in group I and 42 (26.3%) in group II. Most of group I were transient loss, and there was no postoperative hearing loss. However, in group II, transient loss was found in 32 patients and permanent loss in 10 patients, and permanent loss was observed at a high rate in group II, and there were also 5 patients with hearing loss after surgery (Table 3.4).

BAEPs cannot accurately know the anatomy location of each wave, but wave I is known as cochlear organ, and wave III is known as a superior olivary complex of low pons [6]. Therefore, the change from wave I is estimated to occur when the distal part of the cochlear organ and CN VIII are damaged, and the change from wave III is assumed to be the change that occurs mainly when the MVD sinking REZ is damaged.

Changes from wave I or changes from wave III all indicate damage to CN VIII, but if the change from wave III is due to damage from REZ, since REZ does not have myelin, it is relatively more fatal damage to CN VIII when damaged in this area.

According to the results of the study, even though the waveform change occurred in group I, after the main procedure, the wave V latency was almost similar to that of the base data, and most recovered well. However, in group II, most of the

bodies that were still extended beyond the base data did not recover well, and the surgery was completed [9].

3.3.1   Conclusion

When BAEP wave V latency change occurs, it is recommended to perform analysis by dividing into whether it has been extended from wave I (group I) or from wave III ($\geq$0.5 ms) (group II). In particular, if it is extended from wave III ($\geq$0.5 ms), it can be predicted whether the BAEP wave will seriously change in the future and can be very effective in preventing hearing loss after surgery.

3.4   The Operation Ended with BAEP Loss, and the Patient's Hearing Is Normal After the Operation. Why Is That?

Relationship between BAEP loss and postoperative patient hearing

When the BAEP waveform is externally influenced, the waveform changes. So, we are trying to make sure that there is no change in hearing after surgery by observing the change in waveform during surgery. The generally known BAEP warning criteria are wave V latency 1 ms delay and amplitude with a 50% decrease [1, 2]. It is known that if these criteria are met, hearing problems may occur after surgery. However, there are cases in which the patient's hearing is normal after the operation, although the waveform was lost during the operation, the operation was not recovered, and the operation was ended. If so, let's look at why this phenomenon exists.

In a patient who suffered all loss of vascular circulation damage without wave I during surgery, there has never been a case of normal hearing after surgery. However, in the case where the wave I was maintained and the waveform was lost and the patient could not recover until the end of the surgery, we experienced a case where the hearing ability was the same as before the surgery in more than half of the patients (Fig. 3.19).

In the main procedure, when the cochlear nerve is weakly damaged by the brain retractor or suction tip, the waveform changes in latency and amplitude of wave V. The latency change gradually progresses little by little, and the change in amplitude is observed to decrease by 50% or more between 10 and 20 s much faster than the change in latency. If it is damaged a little more severely, wave I remains the same, and the rest of the waveform is lost. Although the recovery time varies depending on the degree of damage, there are cases where the waveform is lost and then recovered immediately, and in some cases, recovery is near the end of the surgery after 20 min or more has elapsed after the waveform is lost (Fig. 3.20).

We think there will be some very late recovery. In other words, it is presumed that they did not recover until the operation was completed and recovered after that.

If the waveform is not rapidly lost during surgery and changes in latency and amplitude are observed little by little but eventually the waveform is lost while remaining wave I, it is not a serious injury. There is no change in hearing in more than half of the patients. Even if there is a change in hearing, there are many cases of partial HL at the level of low-frequency HL (Fig. 3.21).

However, if there is no change in latency and amplitude of the waveform during surgery and if there is a sudden loss, most of the waveforms do not recover and total HL of hearing after surgery is often developed.

If the waveform was lost during surgery and could not be recovered and the operation was terminated, wave I was well-observed, the loss of the waveform during surgery did not occur rapidly, changes in latency and amplitude were observed slightly, and then the waveform was lost due to further progression. Since there may be no change in hearing afterward, it would be better to use steroids such as Solumedrol to help recover.

Fig. 3.19 BAEP loss occurred after Teflon insertion, and surgery was completed without recovery

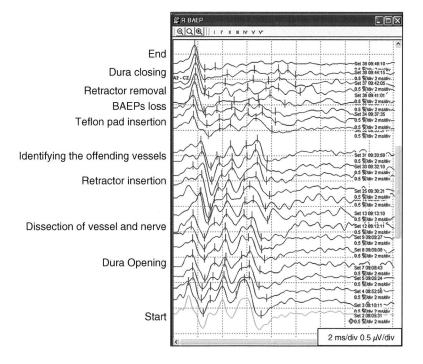

Fig. 3.20 BAEP loss occurred after Teflon insertion, the retractor was immediately removed, and warm saline irrigation gradually recovered the waveform and was well-observed until the end of the surgery

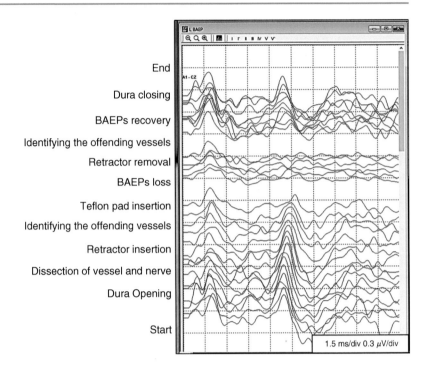

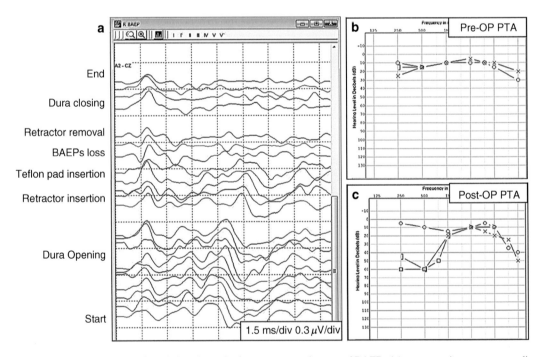

Fig. 3.21 When BAEP waveform is lost due to brain retractor, stack wave of BAEPs (**a**), preoperation pure tone audiometry (**b**), postoperation pure tone audiometry (**c**)

3.5 The Operation Ended with BAEP's Transient Loss and the Patient's Hearing Loss After the Operation. Why Is That?

Relationship between BAEP transient loss and postoperative hearing loss

3.5.1 Permanent Delayed HL

If the body surgery where the BAEP waveform is well-observed is complete, your hearing after surgery is always normal.

If the surgery is not terminated due to the loss of waveform but if the hearing problem occurs after the surgery, it is necessary to check for complex complications. In this case, vascular circulation damage occurs very late.

Even if the BAEPs were observed well during the main procedure, the waveform is rarely lost after the dura is closed later. In this case, it is observed as a waveform that disappears without wave I. The patient is accompanied by problematic complications not only in total HL but also in the vestibular system complaining of severe dizziness. And there is also a case of partial HL, but most of the time high-frequency HL occurs (Fig. 3.22).

If traumatic mechanical damage occurs several times in the main procedure and there are several changes in latency and amplitude of the BAEP waveform wave V, it is important to try to recover to normal sufficiently. This is because in these cases, vascular circulation damage is often delayed. We were relieved because the main procedure was over, and the waveform returned to normal in surgery where severe changes in the waveform due to the brain retractor were observed several times, but there have been several cases of BAEP all loss when the dura was closed and the surgery was almost finished. So, I opened the dura again, administered papaverine, and finished the surgery again after the waveform recovered. In this case, the patient's hearing after surgery was the same as before surgery (Fig. 3.23). In this way, it is important to keep in mind that even if the waveform changes

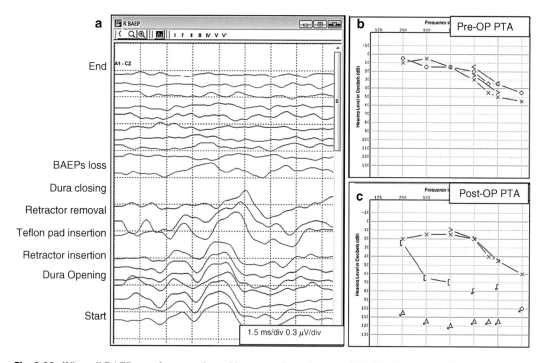

Fig. 3.22 When all BAEP waveforms are lost without wave I, stack wave of BAEPs (**a**), preoperation pure tone audiometry (**b**), postoperation pure tone audiometry (**c**)

Fig. 3.23 BAEP loss occurs after closing the dura, opening the dura again, and restoring the BAEP wave by administering papaverine

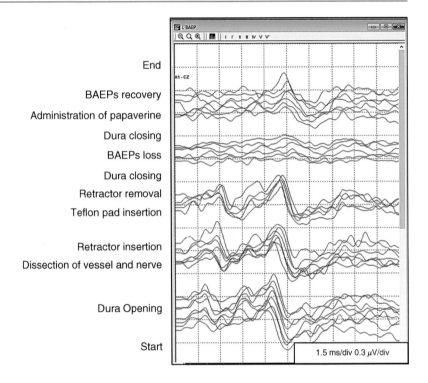

End

BAEPs recovery

Administration of papaverine

Dura closing

BAEPs loss

Dura closing

Retractor removal

Teflon pad insertion

Retractor insertion

Dissection of vessel and nerve

Dura Opening

Start

1.5 ms/div 0.3 µV/div

and recovers during surgery, the waveform change may occur again after the main procedure, and it is very important to observe whether there is any change in the waveform by performing the BAEP test until the operation is completed.

3.5.2   Transient Delayed HL

Delayed HL is a very rare phenomenon in patients with hemifacial spasm. In patients with the same hearing ability as before surgery, sensorineural hearing loss may occur after an average of 22 days after surgery, and high-dose corticosteroid treatment may result in cure after an average of 45 days after surgery. Five patients experienced these patients, and when examining the BAEP waveforms of the patients during surgery, all patients had prolonged wave I–V inter-peak latency and recovered [10].

Although changes in BAEP waveform during surgery vary, the extension of waves I–III inter-peak latency in particular increases the probability of waveform loss during surgery and does not

recover waveform during surgery, given the pre-warning sign (Sect. 3.3). In particular, it should be borne in mind that sensorineural hearing loss may occur suddenly after maintaining normal hearing after surgery (Fig. 3.24).

To define HL, we conduct pure tone audiometry (PTA) and speech discrimination scoring (SDS). PTA and SDS are performed on all patients prior to surgery, and both tests are repeated 7 days after surgery. The average PTA thresholds for 500, 1000, 2000, and 4000 Hz were calculated. We determined postoperative HL status by using most reliable the Association of Otolaryngology–Head and Neck Society (AAO–HNS) classification system (1995).

Postoperative HL (class C/D) was defined as PTA > 50 dB and/or SDS < 50% within the speech frequency range.

During preoperative hearing evaluations, patients with preoperative HL (classes C and D) were excluded from the analysis.

Patients with postoperative HL were classified depending on the frequency of PTA indicating HL as follows: low-frequency HL, high-frequency HL, and total-frequency HL.

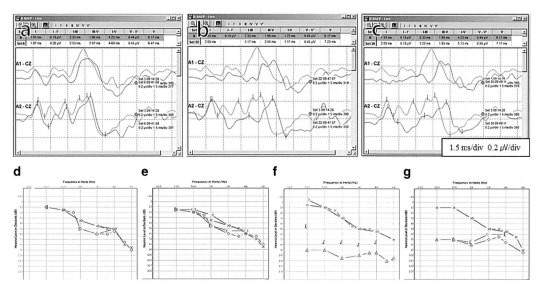

Fig. 3.24 During the operation, initially, brainstem auditory evoked potential (BAEP) showed no unusual findings (**a**). Intraoperatively, sudden prolongation of latency of waves V was observed. There was a prolongation of 1.03 ms, from 6.17 to 7.20 ms (**b**). BAEP findings improved to some extent before the end of the surgery (**c**). Preoperatively, pure tone audiometry and speech discrimination tests yielded normal results (**d**). On postoperative day 3, the patient had normal hearing test results and was discharged from the hospital (**e**). On postoperative day 22, the patient complained of hearing difficulty, and tests confirmed high-frequency sensorineural hearing loss. Corticosteroid treatment was prescribed (**f**). Four months after the operation, hearing function had improved to the preoperative level (**g**)

Fig. 3.25 Association of Otolaryngology–Head and Neck Society (AAO–HNS) classification system (*WRS* word recognition score grading scale)

Hearing Class	PTA Hearing Level (dB)	WRS (%)
A	≤30	≥70
B	>30, ≤50	≥50
C	>50	≥50
D	any level	<50

Low-frequency HL was defined as PTA > 50 dB at 500 and 1000 Hz; high-frequency HL was defined as PTA > 50 dB at 2000 and 4000 Hz. Total-frequency HL was defined as PTA > 50 dB at all measured frequencies [11, 12] (Fig. 3.25).

3.6   Can BAEP Change Occur After the Main Procedure Is Over?

Delayed BAEP change

In general, the section in which waveform change occurs most often occurs during the main procedure. If you think about the reason why, when the flocculus is retracted using a brain retractor, the wave V latency is extended by more than 1 ms, and the amplitude is suddenly decreased by more than 50%. After the main procedure is over and the brain retractor is removed, the waveform gradually begins to recover, and as soon as the dura is closed, the wave V amplitude recovers from 80 to 100%. However, the latency is <1 ms, so surgery is often terminated. In this case, the influence is caused by traumatic mechanical damage, and the waveform changes as soon as it is affected, and when the effect is removed, the waveform is restored over time in proportion to the degree of damage. The general warning criteria we are using is 1 ms delayed; 50% decrease applies here.

However, unusually, there are cases where waveform changes are observed after the main procedure. The waveform was stably observed without any change in the waveform during surgery until the decompression process with Teflon-felt insertion. After the main procedure was finished and the brain retractor was removed, the waveform was suddenly lost. Such cases can be considered by classifying the causes of occurrence into cases of traumatic mechanical damage and vascular circulation damage.

• First, when traumatic mechanical damage occurs slowly and slowly during the main procedure and affects the waveform, the main procedure ends, and the brain retractor is removed. In this case, the traumatic nerve damage accumulated during the main procedure accidentally occurs at the same time when the brain retractor is removed and is observed as a sudden change in the waveform. In fact, as an example of the operation situation, when the operation is performed using the brain retractor during the main

procedure, the BAEP latency may be noticeably extended. Observing the latency that slowly extends little by little and if the wave V latency is extended by more than 1 ms, the examiner informs the surgeon. Surgeon recognizes that the cochlear nerve is affected by the brain retractor, but in the final stage of Teflon insertion, there are cases where the operation is quickly processed without stopping the operation and the brain retractor is removed. In this case, as soon as the brain retractor is removed from time to time, the wave amplitude of BAEPs rapidly decreases by more than 50%. However, in this case, the waveform returns to normal within seconds or minutes.

This is the same phenomenon, but in some cases it may be caused by different effects. At the end of the main procedure, microvessels burst, and bleeding occurred. After bleeding control, the BAEP waveform suddenly disappeared except for wave I. Upon closer examination, it was observed that a hematoma was formed and is giving pressure to the lower part of the cochlear nerve due to bleeding. Therefore, there are cases where the waveform was recovered immediately after removing the hematoma (Fig. 3.26).

Fig. 3.26 BAEP change by hematoma

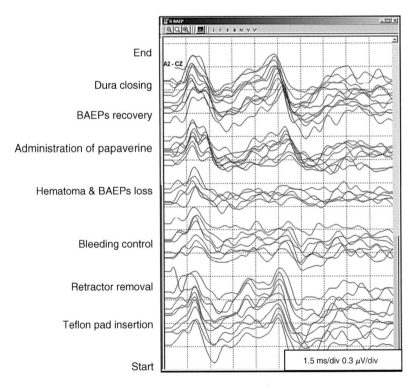

End

Dura closing

BAEPs recovery

Administration of papaverine

Hematoma & BAEPs loss

Bleeding control

Retractor removal

Teflon pad insertion

Start

1.5 ms/div 0.3 μV/div

- Second, it is the change of waveform due to vascular circulation damage. Wave V is observed well during the main procedure without changes in latency and amplitude (Phase I and II steps are not observed), and then the reproducibility of the waveform suddenly disappears. In these cases, both the surgeon performing the surgery and the examiner performing the examination may think the test was measured incorrectly. If the waveform at this time is explained in more detail, the state of the waveform swaying like dancing is observed without the observation of the I, III, and V waveforms of the BAEP wave. In this case, the inspectors may think that the electrode is missing or caused by external artifacts, so they may be left unattended and continued. Waveform reproducibility is abruptly disappeared, and the shape is similar to the artifact as if the electrode is missing. It is observed with a much larger amplitude than the existing waveform for a while and then stabilized with the reproducibility of the waveform. And then BAEPs are observed as wave loss and do not recover until the end of the surgery (Fig. 3.27).

If there is a change in the morphology of the BAEP waveform, it is because a disorder occurs in the vascular circulation. If a problem occurs in the labyrinthine artery, which directly affects the Cochlear nerve, the reproducibility of the waveform is severely lost, and a large-amplitude waveform is observed for a while as if the waveform dances. When a problem occurs in a very small blood vessel such as a perforator, the BAEPs waves I, III, and V are maintained and the reproducibility of the waveform is observed for a while without a little. In this case, a vasodilator such as papaverin should be administered to smooth the vascular circulation flow of the surrounding blood vessels. Otherwise, if left unattended, a loss of total wave that is not observed with wave I is observed, and after surgery, patients become deaf patients complaining of overall disorders of the vestibular system.

To explain the actual surgical situation as an example, it was observed that vasospasm occurred, while decompression of the artery that appears to be a labyrinthine artery from AICA during the main procedure. As this occurred, the waveform was lost. Because the reproducibility of the waveform suddenly disappeared, we thought it was an artifact and could not save the inspection waveform. So in Fig. 3.28, only BAEP wave loss was measured as a stack wave. The waveform was recovered because I was irrigation with a warm saline while waiting for the waveform to recover for about 5 min using papaverin. There was no change in hearing after surgery.

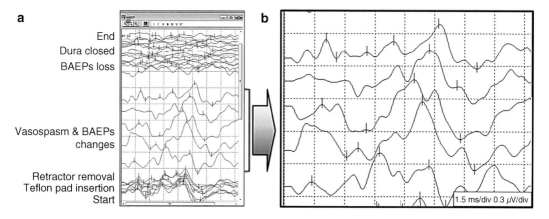

Fig. 3.27 BAEPs change waveform in vascular circulation damage. Stack wave of BAEPs (**a**), focus on vascular circulation damage wave (**b**)

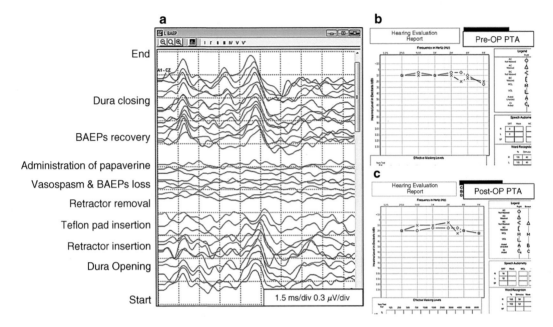

Fig. 3.28 BAEP waveform loss and recovery due to vasospasm, stack wave of BAEPs (**a**), preoperation pure tone audiometry (**b**), postoperation pure tone audiometry (**c**)

3.7 Significance Wave I in BAEPs

The loss of the BAEP waveform is very closely related to the postoperative hearing loss. The change in the BAEP waveform in the main procedure during surgery is traumatic mechanical damage, and the change is reflected in the waveform as soon as the cochlear nerve is damaged. In addition, the effect of vascular circulation damage affects the BAEP waveform in a delayed manner as it takes some time to affect the cochlear nerve because blood circulation is not smooth [13]. In rare cases, the response was measured very slowly, and we also experienced a case where the well-observed waveform without any change during the main procedure was lost after closing the dura. Therefore, we should not neglect that the main procedure for the BAEP test in MVD surgery is over and should be monitored continuously until the end of the surgery.

We can distinguish traumatic mechanical damage or vascular circulation damage by the shape of the waveform. When traumatic mechanical damage is severely affected, BAEP wave loss

occurs, but wave I is always present. In BAEP waveforms of patients with hearing disturbance caused by brain tumor, wave I is present, and latency delayed or amplitude decrease of the remaining waveforms, wave III or V, is similar. In other words, the presence of wave I in the BAEP waveform means that the ability to transmit sound to the cochlear is normal and that there is a problem in the process from the cochlear nerve to the brainstem. In fact, when examining the postoperative hearing status of patients whose wave I was present and all other waveforms were lost, most cases showed only hearing loss or partial HL (Fig. 3.29).

However, in the case of vascular circulation damage, a waveform with no representation is suddenly observed without extending or decreasing wave V, and all waveforms are lost without even wave I. This means that the vestibular cochlear system was all affected overall. In this way, BAEP wave all loss was observed, the surgery was completed without recovery, and the symptoms after surgery were very serious and varied. HL is naturally accompanied, and tinnitus, dizziness, and hoarseness are observed together (Fig. 3.30).

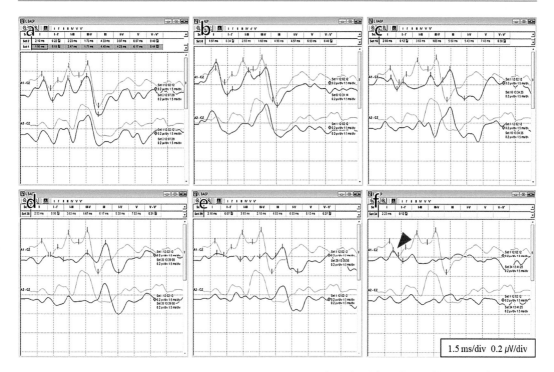

Fig. 3.29 Wave change pattern of traumatic mechanical damage. When the waveform is lost, wave I is always observed (**f**). Before dura open (**a**), after dura open (**b**), retractor insertion (**c**), Teflon pad insertion (**d**), retractor removal (**e**), after dura closed (**f**)

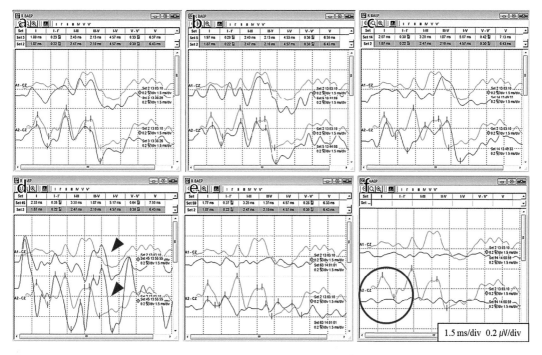

Fig. 3.30 Wave change pattern of vascular circulation damage. In particular, the shape of the waveform becomes irregular without reproducibility (**d**), and when waveform is lost, all waveforms are lost without wave I (**f**). Before dura open (**a**), after dura open (**b**), retractor insertion (**c**), Teflon pad insertion (**d**), retractor removal (**e**), after dura closed (**f**)

3.7.1 Conclusion

We have not been able to clarify in which cases vascular circulation damage occurs. It is only known that it is safe to proceed after the recovery to the normal waveform if the incubation period of the BAEP waveform is extended by more than 2 ms in the main procedure stage during surgery and if the amplitude decreases by more than 50%. During surgery, the BAEP waveform decreased by more than 50%, waited for recovery, and then proceeded again, and again, the waveform decreased by more than 50%, waiting for recovery and then repeating the process several times. Artery related to the cochlear nerve vasospasm occurred frequently. Therefore, if traumatic mechanical damage has occurred several times in the main procedure, it is important to try to restore the BAEP waveform sufficiently to normal. In the end, the cause of vascular circulation damage is also due to traumatic mechanical damage in the main procedure.

If wave I exists when the BAEP waveform is lost during surgery, take measures to remove the brain retractor as traumatic mechanical damage or irrigation with a warm saline while waiting while not directly affecting the cochlear nerve. Most recover. However, there is a difference in recovery time depending on how severely the cochlear nerve is affected by external influences. In some cases very severely affected, recovery may not be possible until the operation is completed.

When BAEP waveform is lost during surgery, all loss without even wave I is vascular circulation damage, which occurs after the completion of the main procedure. In many cases, recovery is not possible due to taking of warm saline. Therefore, more aggressive measures should be taken, such as using drugs that can help blood vessels such as papaverine or raising the blood pressure by lowering the patient's head on the surgical bed.

References

1. Guideline eleven: guidelines for intraoperative monitoring of sensory evoked potentials. Am Electroencephalogr Soc J Clin Neurophysiol 1994;11(1):77–87.
2. Society AE. Guideline eleven: guidelines for intraoperative monitoring of sensory evoked potential. J Clin Neurophysiol. 1994;11(1):77–87.
3. Joo BE, Park S, Cho KR, Kong DS, Seo DW, Park K. Real-time intraoperative monitoring of brainstem auditory evoked potentials during microvascular decompression for hemifacial spasm. J Neurosurg. 2016;125:1061–7. https://doi.org/10.1016/j.clinph.2017.12.032.
4. Park SK, Joo B, Lee S, Lee JA, Hwang JH, Kong DS, Seo DW, Park K, Lee HT. The critical warning sign of real-time brainstem auditory evoked potentials during microvascular decompression for hemifacial spasm. Clin Neurophysiol. 2018;129(5):1097–102. https://doi.org/10.1016/j.clinph.2017.12.032.
5. Thirumala PD, Carnovale G, Habeych ME, Crammond DJ, Balzer JR. Diagnostic accuracy of brainstem auditory evoked potentials during microvascular decompression. Neurology. 2014;83(19):1747–52. https://doi.org/10.1212/WNL.0000000000000961.
6. Little JR, Lesser RP, Lueders H, Furlan AJ. Brain stem auditory evoked potentials in posterior circulation surgery. Neurosurgery. 1983;12(5):496–502. https://doi.org/10.1227/00006123-198305000-00003.
7. Sumito Sato MY, Koizumi H, Onozawa Y, Shimokawa N, Kawashima E, Fujii K. Neurophysiological mechanisms of conduction impairment of the auditory nerve during Cerebellopontine angle surgery. Clin Neurophysiol. 2009;120(2):329–35. https://doi.org/10.1016/j.clinph.2008.11.005.
8. Sindou M, Fobé JL, Ciriano D, Fischer C. Hearing prognosis and intraoperative guidance of brainstem auditory evoked potential in microvascular decompression. Laryngoscope. 1992;102(6):678–82. https://doi.org/10.1288/00005537-199206000-00014.
9. Sang-Ku Park M, Joo B-E, Kwon J, Kim M, Lee S, Lee J-A, Park K. The prewarning sign of brainstem auditory evoked potentials during microvascular decompression surgery for hemifacial spasm. Clin Neurophysiol. 2020;Acceptance letter;23:2020.
10. Lee MH, Lee S, Park SK, Lee JA, Park K. Delayed hearing loss after microvascular decompression for hemifacial spasm. Acta Neurochir. 2019;161(3):503–8. https://doi.org/10.1007/s00701-018-3774-7.
11. American Academy of Otolaryngology-Head and Neck Surgery Foundation I. Committee on hearing and equilibrium guidelines for the evaluation of hearing preservation in acoustic neuroma (vestibular schwannoma). Otolaryngol Head Neck Surg. 1995;113(3):179–80. https://doi.org/10.1016/S0194-5998(95)70101-X.
12. American Academy of Otolaryngology-Head and Neck Surgery Foundation. Committee on hearing and equilibrium guidelines for the evaluation of results of treatment of conductive hearing loss. Otolaryngol Head Neck Surg. 1995;113(3):186–7. https://doi.org/10.1016/S0194-5998(95)70103-6.
13. Joo BE, Park S, Lee MH, Lee S, Lee JA, Park K. Significance of wave I loss of brainstem auditory evoked potentials during microvascular decompression surgery for hemifacial spasm. Clin Neurophysiol. 2020;131(4):809–15. https://doi.org/10.1016/j.clinph.2019.12.409.

4.1 Is It Okay If the LSR Is Not Lost During Surgery?

It is known that loss of LSR during MVD surgery in hemifacial spasm patients means that the separation of facial nerves and blood vessels is well done [1–9]. However, there are cases where they are not lost during surgery and remain unchanged [10]. LSR's latency, amplitude, and shape were all unchanged from the beginning of the operation to the end of the operation. When the patient's postoperative state was observed, the patient's spasm was unexpectedly cured and the patient's satisfaction was high. However, there were very few cases where facial tremors remained the same as before surgery. So, if the LSR is not lost during surgery, it will be best to do a 360-° decompression around the offending site.

Contrary to the case in which LSR is not lost during surgery, the offending vessel may spontaneously separate from the facial nerve as the dura is opened and the cerebellum sunken down in the CSF drain state. Even if the LSR is lost in this way, a wide 360° decompression around the offending site will be required.

If the LSR response does not change at all despite all surgical procedures, additional irradiation and/or decompression are usually performed during surgery to relieve all vascular compression of the facial nerve [11, 12]. However, this method is not recommended because hearing loss or facial paralysis may occur after extensive additional surgery is performed on the surgical site for the purpose of loss of LSR. According to one study, when LSR is lost during surgery, more than 90% of the spasm is resolved after surgery. However, even if it is not lost, it is not a bad thing. Even if it is not lost, it is said that no further action will be taken [9].

We tested both the spasm side and the opposite face to determine if the LSR was a test specific to HFS. LSR is a very specific test for HFS, and it is a test that can be applied very usefully during surgery, considering that no LSR has ever been measured on a normal face that does not shake even after testing more than 1000 people [1–3, 5, 6, 13]. However, there are studies showing that there are many patients with good outcomes after surgery even if they are not lost during surgery [2–5, 14]. The reason for this is that it takes months or years to normalize the excitability of the facial motor nuclei, which causes facial spasms, and the period for normalization is different depending on the severity and duration of spasm symptoms.

In summary, if LSR is not lost during surgery, do not cause facial nerve paralysis or auditory nerve disorders by excessively excessive surgical measures to ensure that the LSR is lost. It is recommended to perform extensive decompression around the offending site and complete the surgery.

4.2   Is There Any HFS Where LSR Is Not Measured?

Learn about five cases where LSR measurement is not possible.

In our experience, the preoperative LSR measurement rate in HFS patients is 88.1%, and the intraoperative LSR measurement rate is 86.2% [15].

The reason why the LSR measurement rate is lower in the intraoperative examination than in the preoperative examination is that when the depth of muscle relaxation of the anesthesia is shallow during the operation, the patient's anesthesia is not maintained, and the LSR measurement cannot be performed due to awakening. This is because, if the measurement was very small below 10 µV, the measurement could not be performed due to the effect of muscle relaxants during surgery. Due to the influence of muscle relaxants during surgery, the amplitude of the LSR test waveform during surgery was measured to be an average of about 100 µV smaller than that of the preoperative test [15]. In some cases, LSR measurement was not possible even if the same area as the LSR area measured before surgery was not stimulated during surgery.

Therefore, it is a good idea to take a picture of the area where LSR is well measured in the patient before surgery and then install the electrode in the same area during surgery (Figs. 4.1 and 4.2).

Let's look at five cases where the LSR side is not smooth during preoperative examination and surgery.

- First, there are obvious symptoms of shaking on the face, but there are cases where it is difficult to observe the waveform when LSR is measured. If the examination is performed while mapping the facial nerve branch very closely and at intervals of 1 mm, there are cases where LSR is measured only at a specific intensity and is very narrow. In this case, when the stimulator is removed from the face and the test is attempted at the same area for the first time, the LSR measurement is not immediately performed, and the measurement site must be searched in detail. In most cases, measurements were not possible. If the range of the facial nerve branch where LSR is measured is very narrow, it may not be measured during surgery.
- Second, there are cases where the LSR can be measured about once after testing ten times. Even if the stimulation intensity is adjusted in various ways and the stimulation site is also applied in several places, the LSR is sometimes

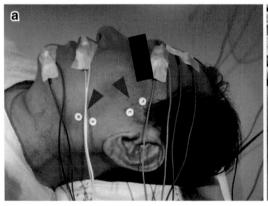
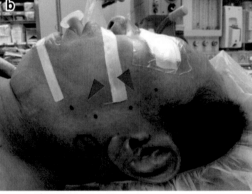

Fig. 4.1 The optimal stimulation site found in the preoperative examination (**a**) and the picture marked on the same area during surgery (**b**)

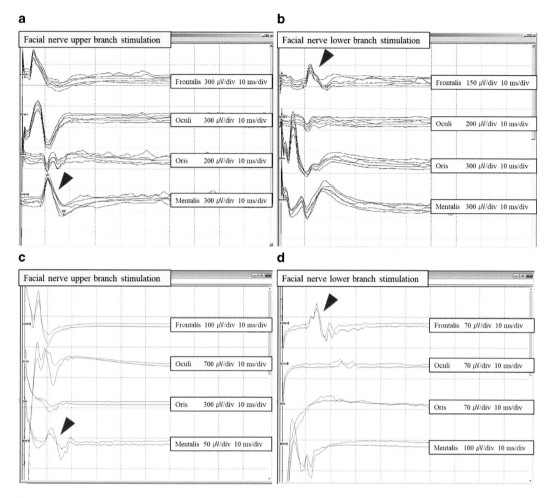

Fig. 4.2 Preoperation upper stimulation LSR, amplitude 495.11 µV (**a**), preoperation lower stimulation LSR, amplitude 114.17 µV (**b**), operation upper stimulation LSR, amplitude 18.64 µV (**c**), operation lower stimulation LSR, amplitude 76.79 µV (**d**)

measured very occasionally. Even in this case, LSR may not be measured during surgery.

- Third, the LSR amplitude is measured too small. In this case, since the amplitude decreases when using a muscle relaxant during surgery, even if it is observed with reproducibility in the preoperative examination, a very small waveform of about 10 µV may not be measured during surgery.
- Fourth, the LSR may not be measured for a few months after the onset of spasm or in patients with very weak spasm. In this case, it is difficult to recommend surgery. This is because LSR measurement will not be possible even during surgery, and LSR help cannot be obtained during surgery.

- Fifth, in patients with hemifacial spasm, it is observed that one eye and around the mouth are occasionally shaking. However, a very severe patient can keep their eyes closed because they are constantly shivering and sometimes open their eyes when they do not shake. In cases where such severe tremors persist, the facial muscles are shaking without rest in the preoperative examination, and the artifacts caused by spasm are mixed more severely than the response from electrical stimulation, so LSR measurement may not be possible. However, since the anesthesia is performed during surgery, LSR measurement is very smooth.

In this way, knowing that there are cases where LSR cannot be measured before or during surgery, if LSR measurement is not successful, it is hoped that the stimulation intensity is increased too much to prevent damage to the facial nerve.

4.3 LSR Was Lost During Surgery, and It Is Measured Again After the Main Procedure. What Does It Mean?

Learn about the seven patterns of LSR loss.

After Teflon insertion, the LSR is lost, so it is determined that the operation has been stably performed, and the LSR is sometimes measured again during the process of ending the operation. In this case, the dura was opened again, and the position of the Teflon entered during the main procedure was finely adjusted, or the operation was just finished (Fig. 4.3). In this case, the

patient had a normal spasm cure after surgery. If so, let's think about why the lost LSR was measured again.

Let's look at the seven patterns in which LSR is lost during surgery.

- First, it is lost immediately after Teflon insertion. These patterns are the most common. It can give you confidence that the operation has been reliably well done.
- Second, it is lost only by touching the offending vessel before insertion of the Teflon. This pattern can be confusing because the LSR is measured and then suddenly disappears and then repeats. In this case, the LSR can be immediately informed as it is observed, giving confidence that the surgical site has been found well.
- Third, after Teflon insertion, LSR is observed as it is for a while and then gradually disappears. If it is lost very late, the dura may be closed and lost.
- Fourth, after Teflon insertion, the LSR waveform is observed once or twice during the ten tests. In this case, you will be worried about how to inform. This case is also similar to the

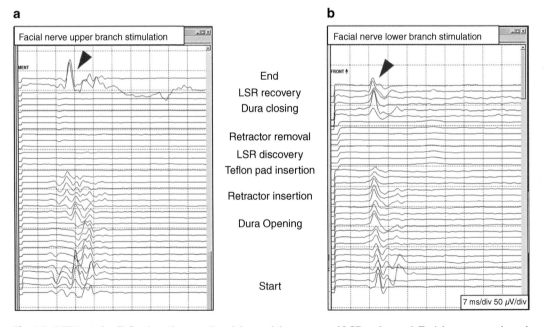

a

Facial nerve upper branch stimulation

b

Facial nerve lower branch stimulation

End
LSR recovery
Dura closing

Retractor removal
LSR discovery
Teflon pad insertion

Retractor insertion

Dura Opening

Start

7 ms/div 50 µV/div

Fig. 4.3 LSR lost after Teflon insertion was closed dura and then measured LSR reobserved. Facial nerve upper branch stimulation (**a**), facial nerve lower branch stimulation (**b**)

Fig. 4.4 Loss of LSR during surgery is a very important indicator. However, it is still not well-known that there are seven different patterns of LSR loss. LSR lost during surgery is often remeasured temporarily

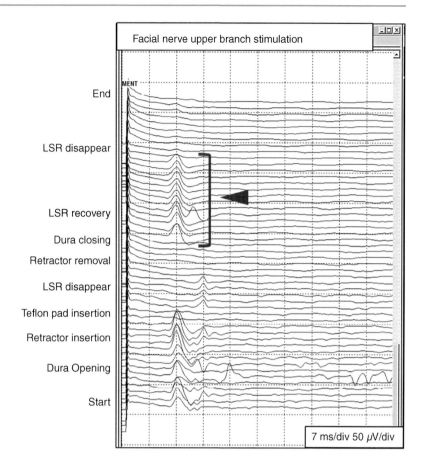

case where it disappears gradually, and the frequency at which LSR is observed decreases over time and eventually disappears completely.

- Fifth, after Teflon insertion, the amplitude of the waveform becomes slightly smaller. In some cases, the amplitude decreases and then becomes smaller and then disappears, and in some cases, the amplitude decreases and is maintained until the operation is completed (discussed in detail in Sect. 4.4).

- Sixth, the shape of LSR changes after Teflon insertion. As the latency and amplitude are changed, the LSR of a completely different shape is measured rather than the original shape. Over time, the modified LSR is also lost (discussed in detail in Sect. 4.5).

- Seventh, it is lost after dura open. It occurs because the offending artery is decompression by itself as the cerebellum sunken down by the CSF drain.

If the LSR lost after Teflon insertion is measured again, it can be confusing. The important thing is that even if there is any change during the operation, it can be considered that the operation was successful as long as it disappears before the end of the operation (Fig. 4.4). In some cases, the LSR is temporarily lost after being measured again, and in some cases, the LSR is slowly lost after Teflon insertion. It should be considered that there are cases where LSR is not always lost immediately after Teflon insertion.

Considering the above seven patterns in which LSR is lost, the case where the LSR lost by Teflon insertion during surgery closes the dura and is measured again is considered to be another type of the fourth pattern. I think it is similar to the case where it disappears slowly or the case where the measured frequency decreases significantly and then disappears. In other words, I think that the LSR is not immediately lost after decompression but is intermittently measured and then lost.

Measurements were made again at the end of the surgery, but I think the LSR would have been lost if the measurements were taken a little longer after the surgery was completed. This is because the spasm was cured in all patients in this case after surgery.

We think as follows.

If there is a change in the LSR response during the main procedure during the surgery, you can think that the offending site has been found well. If the LSR is lost after decompression, you can think that the operation is successful even if the LSR is measured again at the end of the surgery.

4.4   After the Main Procedure, the LSR Amplitude Was Only Slightly Reduced. What Does It Mean?

Learn more about the fifth of the seven patterns of LSR loss.

This is a case where the amplitude of the LSR becomes small and does not disappear, making it difficult to determine whether the operation was successful. Even if the LSR is not lost, studies in which the shape change is observed must be lost during surgery, leading to doubt whether it is good [2–4, 9]. In another study, a decrease in LSR amplitude, similar to the complete disappearance of LSR, is associated with favorable outcomes [11, 16] (Fig. 4.5).

According to our study, 96.4% LSR is lost after the main procedure is completed [15]. Looking at the results of various research studies, the loss of LSR during surgery varies from 55.3 to 95% [2, 3, 11, 12, 17–28].

The reason for this variety of observations may be that the relationship between the loss of LSR during surgery in patients with spasm and the well-being of the surgery is not directly proportional. According to a study by delayed cure, it is reported that the longer the severity and duration of the spasm, the more time it takes to be cured [29]. Similar to this phenomenon, the longer the severity and duration of the spasm is,

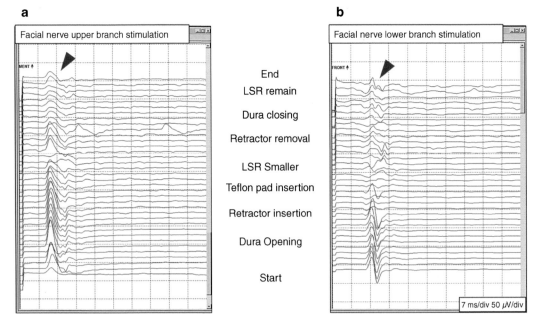

a   b

Facial nerve upper branch stimulation   Facial nerve lower branch stimulation

End
LSR remain

Dura closing

Retractor removal

LSR Smaller

Teflon pad insertion

Retractor insertion

Dura Opening

Start

7 ms/div 50 μV/div

Fig. 4.5 After Teflon insertion, the LSR amplitude decreased and was observed until the operation was completed. Facial nerve upper branch stimulation (**a**), facial nerve lower branch stimulation (**b**)

the more cleanly the LSR is not lost after the main procedure but rather becomes a little smaller, and it is thought that it is measured again after being lost.

We followed up the patients whose LSR amplitude was reduced, and the surgery was terminated without loss, and we found that all patients had no facial tremor symptoms after surgery. Considering the above, I think that the amplitude change of LSR due to Teflon insertion is also significant.

4.5   After the Main Procedure, the LSR Shape Changed and It Is Continuously Measured. What Does It Mean?

Learn more about the sixth of the seven patterns of LSR loss.

LSR, which was well-observed during surgery, sometimes changes shape after Teflon insertion. If the shape changes without disappearing, it becomes embarrassing because you don't know what this phenomenon is. Therefore, even when extensive decompression is performed even around the area considered to be an offending site, the deformed LSR is not lost and can be observed continuously. It is very rare that even if you think it will disappear over time and proceed to the end of the surgery, it does not disappear until the end of the surgery. When we observed the postoperative state of patients who had this phenomenon of changing the shape of the LSR during surgery, all spasm was cured.

The shape of the LSR in this case is different from the shape observed at the beginning of the surgery. There were many cases where the latency was observed to be a little lower, and the cases were observed to be increased more rarely. In addition, there are many cases in which the shape of the waveform is upside down, and the shape of the waveform remains the same, but there is no change only in latency. In many cases,

the amplitude of the waveform was decreased in many cases (Fig. 4.6c), and there were few cases when it was observed to be larger (Fig. 4.6d, e). And most of the LSR was temporarily deformed after Teflon insertion and then disappeared (Fig. 4.6).

It is very difficult to theoretically explain the change in latency and phasic of LSR. However, it is clear that a change occurred in the offending site by Teflon insertion. And even if this happens, the patient showed very good results after surgery. I think that it is the same reason that other studies showed positive results for the change in LSR shape during surgery [2–4].

It is very similar to the above phenomenon, but it is due to a completely different cause, so it is necessary to distinguish it.

When stimulating by increasing the intensity to several times the intensity of the LSR measurement during surgery, the facial nerve innervation varies from person to person, so that the facial nerve in the vicinity is stimulated, and a waveform similar to the LSR is observed [30]. Even in this case, the latency is measured a little faster. However, these waveforms are never lost irrespective of surgery and are not related to the patient's condition after surgery. The reason is completely different from the LSR measurement principle, but care should be taken because there are cases where waveforms are observed very similar to LSR.

4.6   After the Main Procedure, the LSR Amplitude Is Measured Rather Large. What Does It Mean?

In most cases, LSR is lost after Teflon insertion. However, there are cases where it is measured even larger. Sometimes only the amplitude is temporarily measured larger and then disappears. Here, we will look at the case where the shape of the waveform where the LSR is measured as well as the amplitude changes multiphasic and is observed until the end of the operation (Fig. 4.7).

Before and after Teflon insertion, the state of anesthesia remained unchanged, and after Teflon

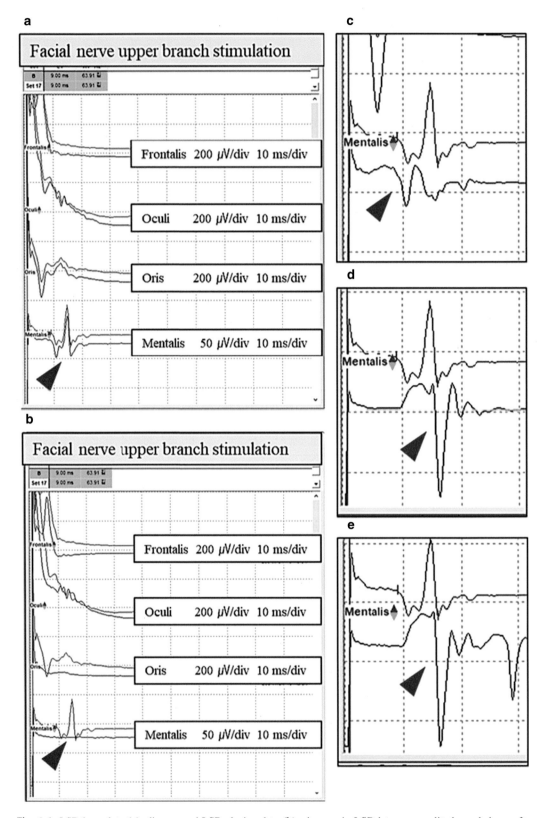

Fig. 4.6 LSR base data (**a**), disappeared LSR closing data (**b**), changes in LSR latency, amplitude, and shape after Teflon insertion (**c, d, e**)

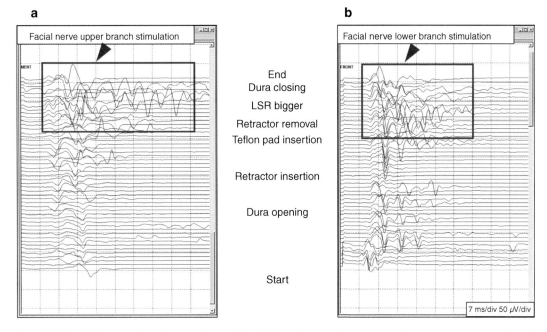

a Facial nerve upper branch stimulation

b Facial nerve lower branch stimulation

End
Dura closing
LSR bigger
Retractor removal
Teflon pad insertion

Retractor insertion

Dura opening

Start

7 ms/div 50 µV/div

Fig. 4.7 After Teflon insertion, the magnitude of the LSR amplitude and the degree of response are measured much stronger

insertion, LSR was measured and measured in multiphasic wave form. When measuring LSR, it was confirmed that no waveform was observed in the free-running EMG, so the LSR waveform was not affected by the mixing of the facial nerve EMG waveform (Fig. 4.8).

Although it is a very rare phenomenon with more than 4000 surgeries, we experienced a case where Teflon was inserted, and LSR was temporarily measured only for a while and then lost. Therefore, I thought it was such a phenomenon, and after completing the Teflon insertion, the LSR was continuously measured, but the operation was terminated. At the second day after the operation, there was no change in the objective findings, but the subjective feeling of the patient seemed to have reduced tremor by 50%. Two months after the operation, the same tremor was observed as before the operation, and at 8 months after the operation, the tremor was more severe than before, so reoperation was considered.

We believe that it is a very dangerous phenomenon for the LSR to be measured larger after Teflon insertion.

4.7 When Measuring LSR, the Electrical Stimulation Intensity Should Be Increased a Little More Than Before. Do I Have to Measure the Electric Stimulation with Each Test?

Learn about the LSR measure the electric stimulation.

When performing electrical stimulation, in order to avoid fatigue or discomfort in the area to be stimulated, high electrical stimulation of 30 mA or more is not used in the preoperative examination when the patient is awake, and LSR is measured between 1 and 30 mA in most patients. Therefore, tests are performed with similar stimulation intensity during surgery. A study on the discomfort and pain of patients due to electrical stimulation to the facial nerve reported that they complained of light flashes, toothaches, and metallic taste before 40 mA [31].

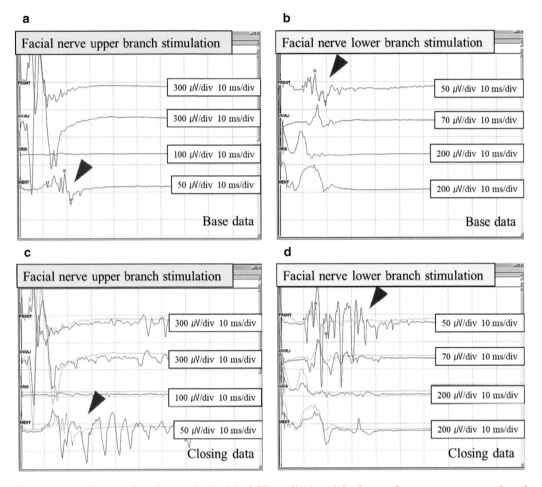

Fig. 4.8 After Teflon insertion, the magnitude of the LSR amplitude and the degree of response are measured much stronger

There is a repeated pulse stimulation method, which is a method that Møller AR and Jannetta PJ measure LSR in two to eight times per second in a row [19, 32] (Fig. 4.9a, b). There is a pulse stimulation method [15](Fig. 4.9c, d). LSR can be observed in both test methods, but in the repeated pulse stimulation method, LSR is not observed for all electrical stimulation, and there is a refractory period, so the reaction is observed mainly at the start site where the electrical stimulation enters. Therefore, the single pulse stimulation test is recommended. The reason is that the LSR test time is very fast, so single pulse stimulation, which can sensitively respond to peripheral surgical manipulations related to the facial nerve, is slightly more sensitive.

The purpose of the LSR test is to evaluate whether the offending site is properly decompressed. Therefore, as explained in Sect. 2.2.1.3, in order to increase the sensitivity of the LSR test, it is easy to discriminate whether it is an offending site to find and test the threshold rather than stimulate it with a strong intensity. As it is LSR lost, it helps to make the operation more smooth.

However, when performing a test that stimulates the threshold like this, the state of the patient's anesthesia depth varies little by little, so the test should be performed while adjusting the intensity of the stimulation. The most basic inspection method is to observe whether or not a waveform with the same shape as the base data is formed. It is true that the LSR waveform is lost when the waveform shape of the facial nerve branch where the stimulus enters is not smaller than the base data. If the LSR is lost and the waveform of the facial nerve branch where the stimulus enters is also reduced, the intensity of the stimulus should be increased to measure the waveform equal to or larger than the base data (Fig. 4.10).

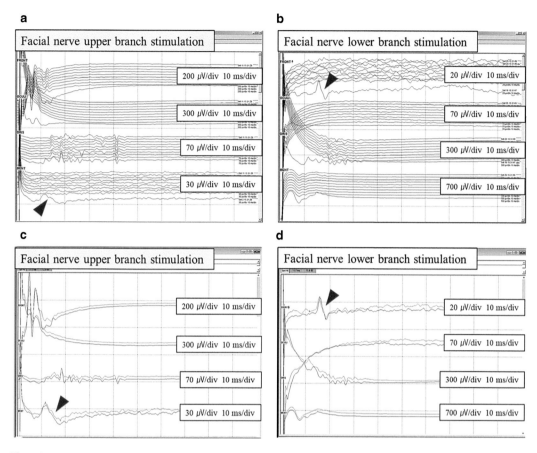

Fig. 4.9 repeated pulse stimulation method (**a, b**) and single pulse stimulation method (**c, d**)

Fig. 4.10 Anesthesia. Because the depth of muscle relaxation is high, neither electrical stimulation artifacts nor responses in the oris and mentalis areas are observed, and the waveforms in both the frontalis and oculi areas where the LSR waveform is measured are lost. (*Green* base data, test active data)

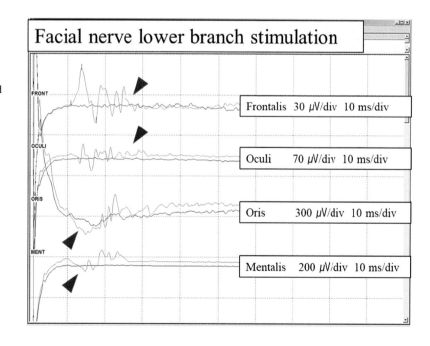

Fig. 4.11 A picture of the loss of LSR measured in mentalis of the lower branch as a stimulus waveform with an active wave larger than the base data was formed when the facial nerve upper branch was stimulated. (*Green* base data, test active data)

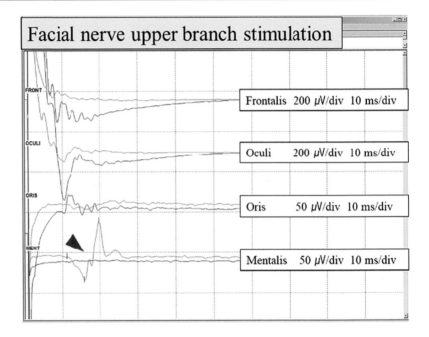

Even if the LSR is lost after the main procedure is finished, it is also important to increase the intensity of the stimulus to determine whether LSR cannot be measured at all intensities (Fig. 4.11).

4.8 Free-Running EMG Waveforms Have Been Continuously Generated Since Teflon-Felt Insertion. In this Case, What Should I Do to Measure LSR?

Learn about optimal muscle relaxant usage during surgery.

In the case of not using a muscle relaxant to facilitate LSR measurement during surgery, we have often experienced a case where the free-running EMG waveform generated during Teflon insertion is continuously generated for a while, making LSR measurement impossible (Fig. 4.12). Alternatively, there was a risky experience of temporarily stopping the operation due to a case of movement of the patient during

surgery, putting the patient to a deep anesthetic depth, and then performing the operation again (Fig. 4.13). So, we studied to find the depth of muscle relaxation anesthesia, where LSR measurements were smoothly performed, and the targets of partial NMB were a TOF count of 2 and a T1/Tc ratio of 50%. LSR measurements were much easier when maintaining anesthesia under these conditions [33].

So we have, for the consistency of AMR monitoring, the response to train-of-four (TOF) stimulation was monitored with maintaining a target of 50% twitch height of the first TOF response from various locations such as ulnar nerve, median nerve, and posterior tibial nerve on the bilateral sides compared to the baseline twitch by the neuromuscular transmission module (M-NMT Module, Datex-Ohmeda, Helsinki, Finland).

LSR can also be measured using muscle relaxants during surgery. However, as the amount of muscle relaxant is increased, the amplitude of LSR is measured to be smaller, and if the muscle relaxant is used strongly, it cannot be measured. Therefore, the anesthesiologist should wait until the LSR measurement is smooth without any further administration of the muscle relaxant, and only the muscle relaxant used at the start of anes-

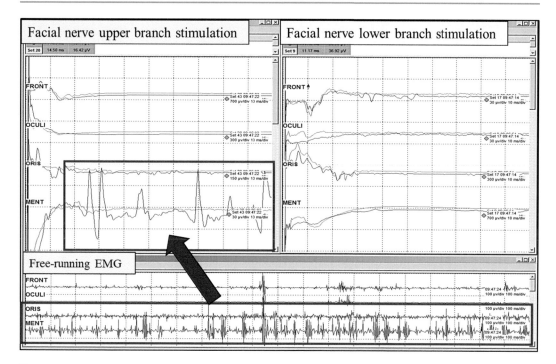

Fig. 4.12 Picture that affects LSR measurement by continuously generating free-running EMG waveform after inserting Teflon

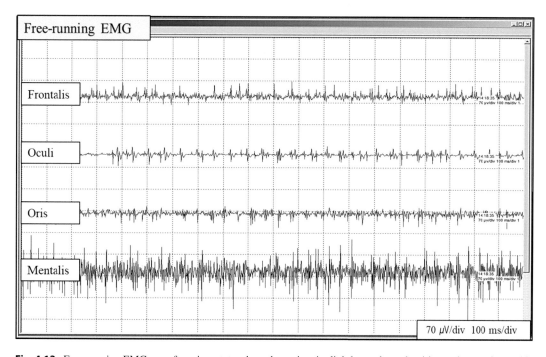

Fig. 4.13 Free-running EMG waveform in a state where the patient is slightly awake and writing an impression on his face because no muscle relaxants are used during surgery

thesia. LSR measurement begins as the effect of the muscle relaxant administered at the beginning of anesthesia begins to gradually weaken.

In order to maintain the muscle relaxation state well at this time, cooperation with the anesthesiologist is requested, and the dosage of the muscle relaxant for maintaining the anesthesia is determined in a small amount. In this muscle relaxation state, only when Teflon is inserted, a temporary waveform is formed in the free-running EMG and immediately disappears, so it does not cause any inconvenience in measuring LSR.

However, the LSR measurement cannot be performed if the anesthesiology does not cooperate to maintain the muscle relaxation state that facilitates the LSR measurement, and if no muscle relaxants are used to make the LSR measurement very smooth, it occurs during Teflon insertion during surgery. There are cases where the free-running EMG waveform continues to occur for a while and rather interferes with the LSR measurement.

Therefore, the use of muscle relaxants enough to measure LSR can ensure stable surgery so that the patient does not wake up during surgery.

It is recommended to use an appropriate muscle relaxant because the free-running EMG waveform is not excessively reacted due to the insertion of Teflon to facilitate LSR measurement.

4.9   When Should the LSR Be Tested During Surgery?

Learn about seven steps of LSR measurement.

LSR is not necessarily lost after decompression but when a lot of CSF flows after dura open, brain sunken down, and facial nerves and offenders are naturally separated and lost [34]. It is important to clearly identify whether the LSR has been lost due to surgical measures.

Otherwise, the surgery could not decompress the facial nerve and offending vessel normally, but the loss of LSR could cause the surgery to be considered successful and to terminate the surgery. Therefore, it is recommended to set the LSR measurement step into seven steps as follows and then inspect it.

- First, it must be measured in the before dura open stage. The measurement of LSR means that the depth of muscle relaxation of the anesthesia is smooth, and in particular, the dura may be lost while opening, so it must be measured before the dura is opened.
- Second is the dura open stage. The dura open stage refers to the time from when the CSF fluid begins to flow through dura incision until the low cranial nerve dissection. During this process, the CSF liquid continues to flow out. In some cases, LSR is lost just before opening all duras and seeing the microscope to proceed with the main procedure (Fig. 4.14).
- Third, it is the before decompression stage. As a stage of performing surgery while looking at the microscope in earnest, it is the stage of examining the relationship between the facial nerve and the offending vessel before Teflon insertion. At this stage, the blood vessel suspected of being an offending vessel is temporarily separated from the facial nerve, and LSR is measured at this time, and it can be confirmed that LSR is lost if it is an offending site (Fig. 4.15).

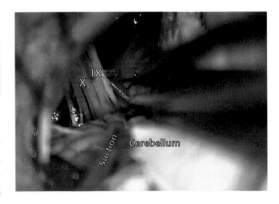

Fig. 4.14 Low cranial nerve dissection stage after dura open

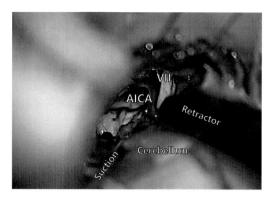

Fig. 4.15 Before decompression step

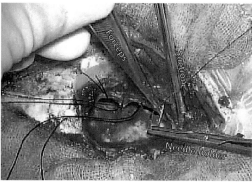

Fig. 4.17 Before dura closed step

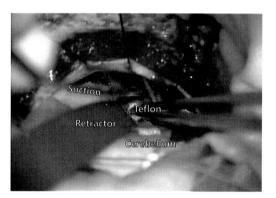

Fig. 4.16 After decompression stage

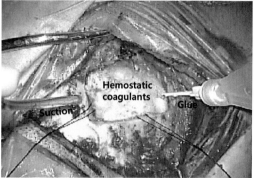

Fig. 4.18 After dura closed step

- Fourth, after Teflon insertion, it is an after decompression stage. Confidence that the main procedure has been completed can be seen as loss of LSR. If Teflon insertion is performed and there is no change in the shape of the LSR, there may be other blood vessels around it. In this case, it is necessary to look closely around the facial nerve, and in some cases, LSR may be lost after decompression of the vein (Fig. 4.16).
- Fifth, before dura closed stage. In some cases, LSR is not lost even after Teflon is inserted. Therefore, it may be lost in the process of closing dura. Therefore, continuously measure LSR to determine the time of loss (Fig. 4.17).
- Sixth, after dura closed stage. Closing the dura is a state in which no further changes occur in the structure of the facial nerve and Teflon, and in this state, you will live your daily life

after surgery. Therefore, measure and observe whether the lost LSR cannot be observed continuously (Fig. 4.18).
- Seventh is the operation end stage. By the end of the surgery, the anesthetic concentration is shallow. This is because the patient has to be awakened soon afterward from anesthesia. Therefore, the measurement of LSR at this stage is the closest to the postoperative state. Therefore, the LSR is finally measured.

While LSR is a very useful test during surgery, we know that it is not always a reliable test [9, 10, 14]. However, the reliability of LSR is still high, and LSR is lost after Teflon insertion in most surgery [1–4, 9, 14]. Therefore, measuring LSR by dividing it into seven steps can help to use it as an index linking the meaning of true LSR and the success of surgery.

References

1. Fernández-Conejero I, Ulkatan S, Sen C, Deletis V. Intraoperative neurophysiology during microvascular decompression for hemifacial spasm. Clin Neurophysiol. 2012;123(1):78–83. https://doi.org/10.1016/j.clinph.2011.10.007.

2. Kiya N, Bannur U, Yamauchi A, Yoshida K, Kato Y, Kanno T. Monitoring of facial evoked EMG for hemifacial spasm: a critical analysis of its prognostic value. Acta Neurochir. 2001;143:365–8. https://doi.org/10.1007/s007010170091.

3. Mooij JJ, Mustafa M, van Weerden TW. Hemifacial spasm: intraoperative electromyographic monitoring as a guide for microvascular decompression. Neurosurgery. 2001;49:1365–71. https://doi.org/10.1097/00006123-200112000-00012.

4. Tobishima H, Hatayama T, Ohkuma H. Relation between the persistence of an abnormal muscle response and the long-term clinical course after microvascular decompression for hemifacial spasm. Neurol Med Chir (Tokyo). 2014;54:474–82. https://doi.org/10.2176/nmc.oa2012-0204.

5. Von Eckardstein K, Harper C, Castner M, Link M. The significance of intraoperative electromyographic Blateral spread in predicting outcome of microvascular decompression for hemifacial spasm. J Neurol Surg B Skull Base. 2014;75:198–203.

6. Hyun SJ, Kong DS, Park K. Microvascular decompression for treating hemifacial spasm: lesion learned from a prospective study of 1,174 operations. Neurosurg Rev. 2010;33:325–34. https://doi.org/10.1007/s10143-010-0254-9.

7. Kondo A. Follow-up results of microvascular decompression in trigeminal neuralgia and hemifacial spasm. Neurosurgery. 1997;40(1):46–51; discussion 51-2. https://doi.org/10.1097/00006123-199701000-00009.

8. Shimizu K, Matsumoto M, Wada A, Sugiyama T, Tanioka D, Okumura H, Fujishima H, Nakajo T, Nakayama S, Yabuzaki H, Mizutani T. Supine no-retractor method in microvascular decompression for hemifacial spasm: results of 100 consecutive operations. J Neurol Surg B Skull Base. 2015;76:202–7. https://doi.org/10.1055/s-0034-1396660.

9. von Eckardstein K, Harper C, Castner M, Link M. The significance of intraoperative electromyographic "lateral spread" in predicting outcome of microvascular decompression for hemifacial spasm. J Neurol Surg B Skull Base. 2014;75(3):198–203. https://doi.org/10.1055/s-0034-1368145.

10. Thirumala PD, Wang X, Shah A, Habeych M, Crammond D, Balzer JR, Sekula R. Clinical impact of residual lateral spread response after adequate microvascular decompression for hemifacial spasm: a retrospective analysis. Br J Neurosurg. 2015;29(6):818–22. https://doi.org/10.3109/02688697.2015.1054351.

11. Haines SJ, Torres F. Intraoperative monitoring of the facial nerve during decompressive surgery for hemifacial spasm. J Neurosurg. 1991;74(2):254–7. https://doi.org/10.3171/jns.1991.74.2.0254.

12. Huang BR, Chang C, Hsu JC. Intraoperative electrophysiological monitoring in microvascular decompression for hemifacial spasm. J Clin Neurosci. 2009;16(2):209–13. https://doi.org/10.1016/j.jocn.2008.04.016.

13. Yang M, Zheng X, Ying T, Zhu J, Zhang W, Yang X, Li S. Combined intraoperative monitoring of abnormal muscle response and Z-L response for hemifacial spasm with tandem compression type. Acta Neurochir. 2014;156:1161–6. https://doi.org/10.1007/s00701-014-2015-y.

14. Hatem J, Sindou M, Vial C. Intraoperative monitoring of facial EMG responses during microvascular decompression for hemifacial spasm: prognostic value for long-term outcome: a study in a 33-patient series. Br J Neurosurg. 2001;15(6):496–9. https://doi.org/10.1080/02688690120105101.

15. Lee S, Park S, Lee JA, Joo BE, Kong DS, Seo DW, Park K. A new method for monitoring abnormal muscle response in hemifacial spasm: a prospective study. Clin Neurophysiol. 2018;129(7):1490–5. https://doi.org/10.1016/j.clinph.2018.03.006.

16. Ishikawa M, Ohira T, Namiki J, Kobayashi M, Takase M, Kawase T, Toya S. Electrophysiological investigation of hemifacial spasm after microvascular decompression: F waves of the facial muscles, blink reflexes, and abnormal muscle responses. J Neurosurg. 1997;86(4):654–61. https://doi.org/10.3171/jns.1997.86.4.0654.

17. Joo WI, Lee K, Park HK, Chough CK, Rha HK. Prognostic value of intra-operative lateral spread response monitoring during microvascular decompression in patients with hemifacial spasm. J Clin Neurosci. 2008;15(12):1335–9. https://doi.org/10.1016/j.jocn.2007.08.008.

18. Neves DO, Lefaucheur JP, de Andrade DC, et al. Are appraisal of the value of lateral spread response monitoring in the treatment of hemifacial spasm by microvascular decompression. J Neurol Neurosurg Psychiatry. 2009;80(12):1375–80. https://doi.org/10.1136/jnnp.2009.172197.

19. Møller AR, Jannetta P. Monitoring facial EMG responses during microvascular decompression operations for hemifacial spasm. J Neurosurg. 1987;66(5):681–5. https://doi.org/10.3171/jns.1987.66.5.0681.

20. Hatem J, Sindou M. Intraoperative monitoring of facial EMG responses during microvascular decompression for hemifacial spasm. Prognostic value for long-term outcome: a study in a 33patient series. Br J Neurosurg. 2001;15(6):496–9. https://doi.org/10.1080/02688690120105101.

21. Sekula RF Jr, Bhatia S, Frederickson AM, et al. Utility of intraoperative electromyography in microvascular decompression for hemifacial spasm: a meta-analysis. Neurosurg Focus. 2009;27(4):E10. https://doi.org/10.3171/2009.8.focus09142.

22. Thirumala PD, Shah A, Nikonow TN, et al. Microvascular decompression for hemifacial spasm: evaluating outcome prognosticators including the value of intraoperative lateral spread response monitoring and clinical characteristics in 293 patients. J Clin Neurophysiol. 2011;28(1):56–66. https://doi.org/10.1097/WNP.0b013e3182051300.

23. Haines SJ, Torres F. Intraoperative monitoring of the facial nerve during decompressive surgery for hemifacial spasm. J Neurosurg. 1991;74(2):254–7.

24. Kong DS, Park K, Shin BG, Lee JA, Eum DO. Prognostic value of the lateral spread response for intraoperative electromyography monitoring of the facial musculature during microvascular decompression for hemifacial spasm. J Neurosurg. 2007;106(3):384–7. https://doi.org/10.3171/jns.2007.106.3.384.

25. Yamashita S, Kawaguchi T, Fukuda M, Watanabe M, Tanaka R, Kameyama S. Abnormal muscle response monitoring during microvascular decompression for hemifacial spasm. Acta Neurochir. 2005;147(9):933–7; discussion 937–938. https://doi.org/10.1007/s00701-005-0571-x.

26. Li J, Zhang Y, Zhu H, Li Y. Prognostic value of intra-operative abnormal muscle response monitoring during microvascular decompression for long-term outcome of hemifacial spasm. J Clin Neurosci. 2012;19(1):44–8. https://doi.org/10.1016/j.jocn.2011.04.023.

27. Huang BR, Chang C, Hsu JC. Intraoperative electrophysiological monitoring in microvascular decompression for hemifacial spasm. J Clin Neurosci. 2009;16(2):209–13.

28. Isu T, Kamamda K, Mabuchi S, Kitaoka A, Ito T, Koiwa M, Abe H. Intra-operative monitoring by facial electromyographic responses during microvascular decompressive surgery for hemifacial spasm. Acta Neurochir. 1996;138(1):19–23; discussion 23. https://doi.org/10.1007/BF01411718.

29. Li MW, Jiang X, Wu M, He F, Niu C. Clinical research on delayed cure after microvascular decompression for Hemifacial spasm. J Neurol Surg A Cent Eur Neurosurg. 2020;81(3):195–9. https://doi.org/10.1055/s-0039-1698461.

30. Katz AD, Catalano P. The clinical significance of the various anastomotic branches of the facial nerve. Report of 100 patients. Arch Otolaryngol Head Neck Surg. 1987;113(9):959–62. https://doi.org/10.1001/archotol.1987.01860090057019.

31. Volk GF, Thielker J, Möller MC, Majcher D, Mastryukova V, Altmann CS, Dobel C, Guntinas-Lichius O. Tolerability of facial electrostimulation in healthy adults and patients with facial synkinesis. Eur Arch Otorhinolaryngol. 2020;277:1247–53.

32. Chuyi Huanga S, Chu H, Dai C, Wu J, Wang J, Zuo H. An optimized abnormal muscle response recording method for intraoperative monitoring of hemifacial spasm and its long-term prognostic value. Int J Surg. 2017;38:67–73. https://doi.org/10.1016/j.ijsu.2016.12.032.

33. Chung YH, Kim W, Lee JJ, Yang SI, Lim SH, Seo DW, Park K, Chung IS. Lateral spread response monitoring during microvascular decompression for hemifacial spasm. Anaesthesist. 2014;63:122–8. https://doi.org/10.1007/s00101-013-2286-3.

34. Kim CH, Kong D, Lee JA, Park K. The potential value of the disappearance of the lateral spread response during microvascular decompression for predicting the clinical outcome of Hemifacial spasms: a prospective study. Neurosurgery. 2010;67(6):1581–8. https://doi.org/10.1227/NEU.0b013e3181f74120.

Cases of Free-Running Electromyography

5.1 How Dangerous Is It to Observe the EMG Waveform During Teflon-Felt Insertion?

Shapes of Free-Running EMG Waveforms

Of course, facial nerve EMG must be measured because it is a surgery that inserts Teflon in the root exit zone of the facial nerve [1, 2]. Looking at the main procedure, in order to prevent facial nerve palsy from occurring as much as possible after surgery, only the offending vessel is separated from the offending site while not touching the facial nerve, and then the Teflon is inserted (Fig. 5.1).

EMG waveforms generated during the Teflon insertion process are largely classified into three types and observed [3].

- First, it is a spike wave. It is observed only once with a waveform similar to an EKG. These waveforms occur when touching the facial nerve very weakly and have no effect on the facial nerve function (Fig. 5.2).
- Second, it is a burst wave. These waveforms are caused by a bunch of spike waves that are gathered together and are caused by weakly touching the facial nerve. In general, it is the most observed waveform when Teflon is

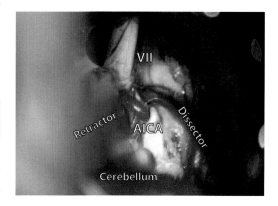

Fig. 5.1 Picture of separating AICA, thought to be an offending vessel affecting the facial nerve, with a dissector

inserted. It is observed only when Teflon is inserted, and not other than that. The amplitude of the burst wave is slightly different depending on the state of the anesthesia's muscle relaxation depth or the patient's facial muscle state, but does not significantly affect the facial nerve function (Fig. 5.3).
- Third, it is a train wave. This waveform is again divided into three types:
  - A-train wave is a high-frequency low-amplitude waveform that causes fatal damage to facial nerve function. A-trains are rhythmic waveforms composed of at least four "spike-like" mono- to triphasic discharges (elements) that start suddenly with typical amplitudes of 100 to

Fig. 5.2 Spike wave

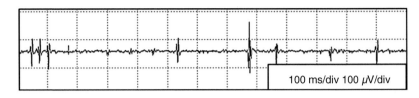

100 ms/div 100 μV/div

Fig. 5.3 Burst wave

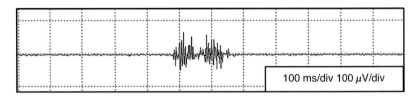

100 ms/div 100 μV/div

Fig. 5.4 A-train wave
≒ high-frequency
low-amplitude

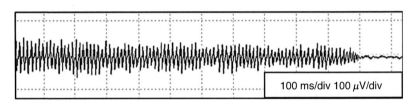

100 ms/div 100 μV/div

Fig. 5.5 B-train wave

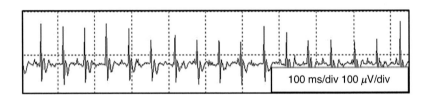

100 ms/div 100 μV/div

200 μV. With the terms of classic nomenclature applied, they soonest resemble "myokymic discharges." The inter-element frequency range for A-trains given in the published classification is 60 to 210 Hz [4]. These waveforms must never be observed during surgery, and facial nerve palsy must be severely generated after surgery (Fig. 5.4).

- B-train wave is a waveform observed by regular and repeated spike wave or burst wave. It occurs when the Teflon is moved from the facial nerve left and right or up and down with fine adjustment after inserting the Teflon. B-trains have been described as a rhythmic or semirhythmic sequence of "elements," which resemble spikes in the Bs-train ("with spikes") or bursts in the Bb-train ("with bursts"). The interval between elements can have a length of up to 500 ms, resulting in a frequency of 2 Hz built by the

single elements. Most subtypes of B-trains resemble "neurotonic discharges" in terms of classic, electrophysiologic nomenclature [3]. It is a very common waveform when inserting Teflon, and it is observed continuously for less than 5 seconds and then disappears (Fig. 5.5).

- C-train wave refers to a condition in which the burst wave is irregular and is directly affected by the facial nerve with high amplitude. The main criterion separating the C-train from the B-train is the loss of a discernible baseline. If such a waveform persists for a long time, facial nerve palsy may occur after surgery, so if it is observed, it is necessary to notify it immediately and take measures so that the waveform is lost (Fig. 5.6).

Burst wave is a waveform that occurs when a nerve is directly touched, and a train wave is a

Fig. 5.6 C-train wave (burst wave가 irregular 하고 high-amplitude)

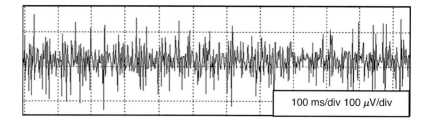

100 ms/div 100 μV/div

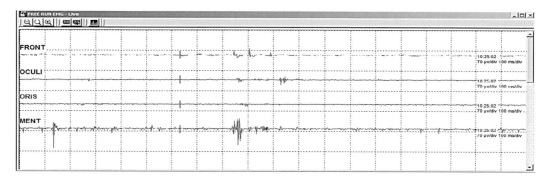

Fig. 5.7 Mild burst wave and spike wave during Teflon insertion

waveform that occurs when a nerve is pulled [5]. Free-running EMG occurs because the facial nerve can be touched or pulled during the Teflon insertion process, and waveforms such as spike and burst waves are observed in a very stable operation. However, when the B-train wave is observed, the surgeon must be informed that the EMG wave is continuously observed weakly, and this report must be made so that the surgeon knows the condition of the facial nerve due to the surgical manipulation.

In particular, when a C-train wave is observed, it is necessary to inform the surgeon that the EMG wave is continuously observed strongly in order to prevent further facial nerve damage. Another way to hear the response of the free-running EMG is through a speaker. If the surgeon is able to hear the free-running EMG sound in real time while performing surgery and the examiner directly communicates the EMG aspect, the facial nerve will be more reliably protected.

In the case of inserting multiple Teflons into a site considered to be an offending site, not all EMG reactions occur every time Teflon is inserted in free-running EMG. In other words, when Teflon is inserted, there may be no or strong free-running EMG reaction. However, in most cases,

LSR is lost after a strong free-running EMG reaction appears, and the site is most often a true offending site. Therefore, if the examiner well expresses the free-running EMG response that occurs during Teflon insertion and cooperates so that the surgeon understands it well, the surgery can proceed well in the right direction, and reoperation will not occur [6].

It is a very common phenomenon that the spike wave of the EMG waveform is observed during Teflon insertion, and then the burst wave is suddenly generated, and the B-train wave is continuously observed for a while (Figs. 5.7 and 5.8). However, if a C-train wave occurs, it is seriously affected, so you need to notify it immediately and take action. If the C-train wave is observed several times, there may be temporary sequelae of facial nerve palsy grade 3 after surgery, so care should be taken.

In free-running EMG, different waveforms of frontalis, oculi, oris, and mentalis are observed in most cases. If a serious waveform is observed in any one place, it is important to immediately inform which waveform has occurred. This is because damage to the facial nerve occurs even when an abnormal waveform is partially generated in the facial nerve.

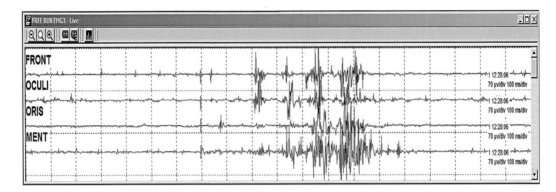

Fig. 5.8 Severe burst wave during Teflon insertion

5.2 After the Teflon-Felt Insertion, the Facial Nerve Is No Longer Touched, But the EMG is Continuously Measured. What Does It Mean?

In the main procedure, the free-running EMG waveform, which only occurs when the facial nerve is touched, sometimes occurs even when it is not touched. These cases are divided into two:

- First, when excessive pressure is applied to the facial nerve. Due to the Teflon insertion, the offending vessel and the facial nerve must be decompressed. If the Teflon is inserted too much, it may be rather compressed. In this case, the free-running EMG waveform is continuously observed as the waveform observed when Teflon insertion is performed, and it can be discriminated that the EMG waveform is observed larger if it touches the offending site. In some cases, it was observed until the dura was closed after the main procedure was finished. In this case, serious facial nerve palsy occurs after surgery, so care should be taken (Fig. 5.9).

- Second, even when the facial nerve activity is very sensitive due to the shallow muscle relaxation of anesthesia, the free-running EMG waveform generated during Teflon insertion may persist for a while and then disappear. In this case, it can be distinguished that the free-

running EMG waveform is observed with a much smaller amplitude than the EMG waveform observed during Teflon insertion (Fig. 5.10). In this way, even after Teflon insertion, if the free-running EMG waveform is observed, it is difficult to determine whether the operation was successful because it interferes with the LSR measurement. Therefore, it is better to set the degree of muscle relaxation to a depth that allows the LSR to be measured rather than to make it unconditionally shallow. Maintaining an appropriate depth of muscle relaxation facilitates observation of the free-running EMG waveform due to Teflon insertion during surgery, enabling the correct evaluation of facial nerve function and allowing LSR measurement immediately after Teflon insertion to facilitate surgery. To make the evaluation smooth.

Looking at the free-running EMG waveform observed during the main procedure, very small spike waves are observed when the offending vessel is separated from the facial nerve (Fig. 5.11a). During Teflon insertion, bursted waveforms are observed (Fig. 5.11b). When fine-tuning the Teflon, which had already been inserted, a bursted waveform was observed again, or a B-train wave was observed (Fig. 5.11c, d). Even if the facial nerve is no longer touched, small spike waves are observed temporarily (Fig. 5.11e), and all waveforms are lost (Fig. 5.11f). This free-running EMG waveform is a pattern of typical waveforms that occur

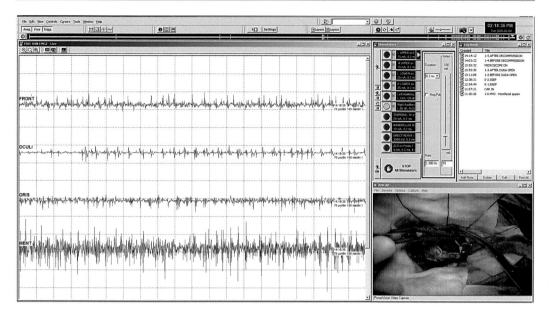

Fig. 5.9 The waveform of the C-train wave is observed from the time of Teflon insertion to the process of the free-running EMG wave being observed until the dura is closed

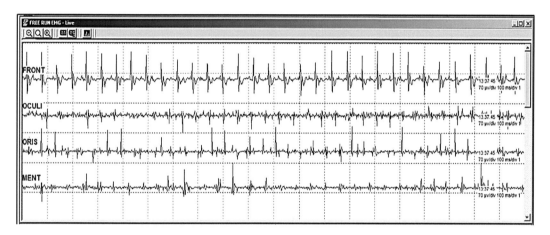

Fig. 5.10 Continuous waveform generated in free-running EMG due to Teflon insertion

during Teflon insertion, and if such a pattern is observed, facial nerve palsy does not occur after surgery.

The degree of damage to the facial nerve due to Teflon insertion is not the type of temporary waveform observed in free-running EMG but whether there is a free-running EMG waveform that is continuously observed even after Teflon insertion is completed, and the shape of the waveform at this time is observed. It is important to do.

If the C-train wave is continuously observed in the free-running EMG even after Teflon insertion is complete, the Teflon insertion is excessive, or the facial nerve is severely affected during the Teflon insertion process. In this case, it is necessary to check whether the effect on the facial nerve is resolved by removing the inserted Teflon or opening the offending vessel. If the C-train wave is lost in the free-running EMG due to this method, it would be a good idea to insert another Teflon shape (Fig. 5.12).

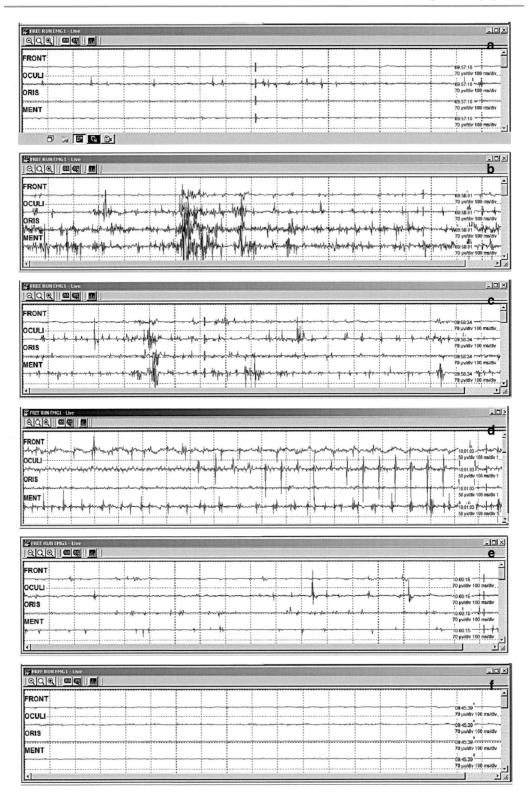

Fig. 5.11 In general, burst waveforms are intensively observed (**a**) during Teflon insertion (**b**), after Teflon insertion (**c**), retractor removal (**d**), before dura closed (**e**), after dura closed (**f**) B-train waves or spiked waveforms are occasionally observed and then disappeared

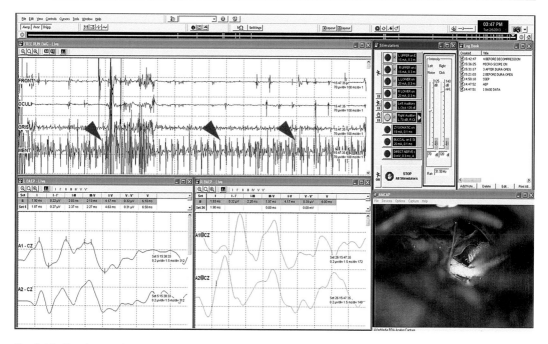

Fig. 5.12 C-train wave in mentalis muscle due to Teflon insertion

5.3   When Saline Irrigation After Main Procedure, EMG Occurs Very Badly. What Does It Mean?

In saline irrigation, free-running EMG generally occurs.

It is difficult to know to what extent the waveform temporarily observed in free-running EMG affects nerves because there is no research report on the method of irrigation or the intensity of saline spraying. However, although the shape of the waveform observed in free-running EMG is very serious, the free-running EMG waveform due to saline irrigation does not seriously affect the facial nerve, as there is no facial nerve palsy after surgery. It is judged to be (Fig. 5.13).

LSR measurement is often impossible due to facial EMG caused by saline irrigation. Therefore, it would be good to make the LSR measurement smooth by making the saline irrigation very weak and little by little so that the free-running EMG does not generate strong waveforms (Fig. 5.14).

Even in the case of cerebellopontine angle tumor, the free-running EMG in the intracranial nerve sometimes causes severe waveforms due to saline irrigation (Fig. 5.15). In addition, C-train wave is observed when intradural saline irrigation is performed in spine tumor (Fig. 5.16).

In particular, when free-running EMG is observed in cold saline irrigation, the latency of BAEPs wave V is prolonged, and the amplitude decreases. In severe cases, BAEP loss may occur temporarily (Fig. 5.17). Therefore, it is recommended to do weak irrigation with a warm saline.

The free-running EMG waveform generated by saline irrigation is observed in the same shape as the waveform generated in direct traumatic nerve damage. Most of them do not occur weakly like spike waves, but very large amplitudes like C-train waves are observed. When the main procedure is over and a large waveform is suddenly observed in the process of closing the dura, it is very surprising. However, compared to the observed waveform of very large amplitude, the patient's condition after surgery is very normal, so there seems to be no association between these waveforms and nerve damage. In other words, although the shape of the waveform generated when direct traumatic nerve damage and the free-running EMG waveform generated by saline irrigation may look similar, it is thought that the

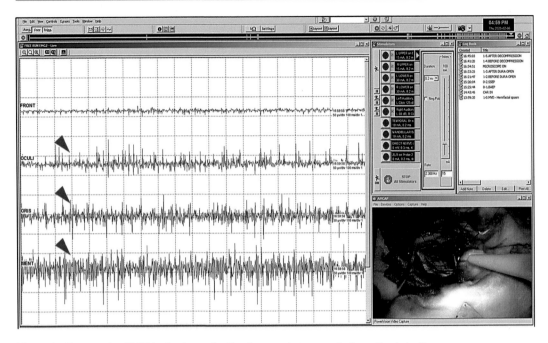

Fig. 5.13 Free-running EMG in the shape of a C-train wave that occurs during saline irrigation

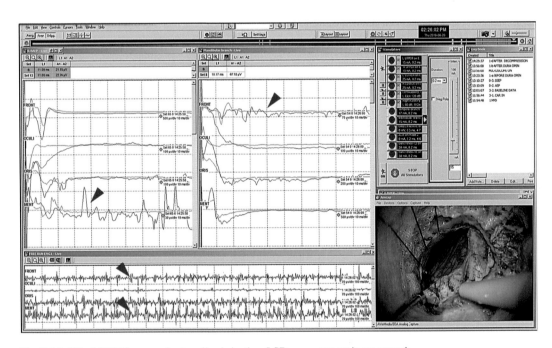

Fig. 5.14 If facial EMG occurs due to saline irrigation, LSR measurement is not smooth

state in which the nerve is actually damaged is completely different.

Looking at the research on free-running EMG, saline contains higher concentrations of Na+ (154 mEq/l) than in lactic solution (130 mEq/l) or aCSF (145.4 mEq/l) So we found that injection of saline activity was more effective in eliciting activity than a lactic solution or aCSF in patients with HFS. There is also a study that suggested [7].

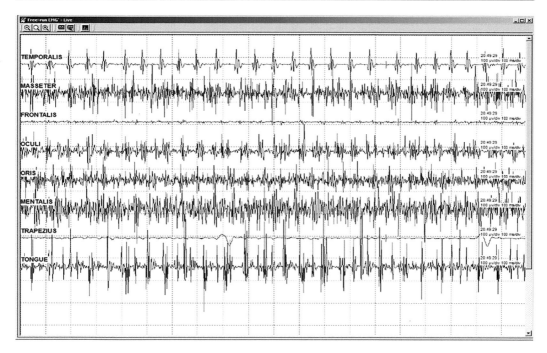

Fig. 5.15 After saline irrigation discharge in skull base surgery

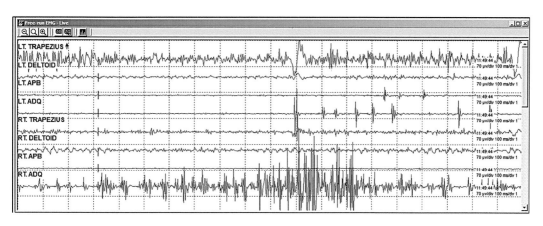

Fig. 5.16 After saline irrigation discharge in spinal cord tumor

5.4 Before Dura Open, the Free-Running EMG Waveform Is Continuously Observed. What Does It Mean?

This is a phenomenon that occurs when the patient's self is alive.

When the muscle relaxation anesthesia is shallow, the patient's spontaneous breathing occurs under normal circumstances, blood pressure rises, and the patient moves. So, because the vital sign changes and the respiration wave changes, the anesthesiologist knows first. However, it often happens that only the free-running EMG waveform changes without any change in any vital sign (Fig. 5.18).

The method of determining whether the patient's muscle relaxation is due to the shallow depth of relaxation is that the amplitude of the free-running EMG waveform is increased by

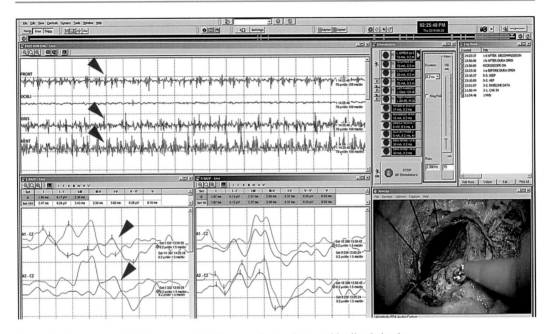

Fig. 5.17 Free-running EMG wave and BAEPs wave change due to cold saline irrigation

performing an electrical stimulation test that causes some pain in the patient. In this state, even if LSR is tested, it is difficult to distinguish between the spread response and the existing EMG.

When the patient's self-EMG occurs due to the shallow relaxation of the anesthesia muscle, the same occurs in the surgery to observe the intracranial nerve and the surgery to remove the tumor to observe the spinal nerve. In general, the train-of-four (TOF) test is considered to be in a relaxed state in which peripheral nerve muscles are activated only when the ratio of T4 and T1 is similar. Therefore, there are cases where anesthesiologists are asked to maintain TOF 4/4. In this case, when the muscle relaxation state is shallow, self EMG often occurs, and when this waveform is observed EMG, it can be mistaken for nerve damage caused by surgical manipulation. It can be misunderstood as a waveform and

mistake it for a nerve path in a path that doesn't actually exist, which can confuse the surgeon performing the operation.

During surgery, if the patient's self is alive and moving, an anesthetic agent is administered through the bolus for the patient's stable vitality. In this case, the self-free-run EMG waveform, which was caused by the shallow depth of muscle relaxation, disappears. However, in MVD surgery, where the main procedure is very short, it becomes difficult to observe the LSR reaction after Teflon insertion, and it becomes difficult to distinguish facial nerve damage. It becomes difficult to judge. Therefore, it is recommended to set the depth of muscle relaxation during surgery to the depth at which the LSR is measured. In general, LSR is measured well enough with a T1/Tc ratio of 50%, and it is considered a very good depth of muscle relaxation because the patient does not wake up slightly from anesthesia [8].

a

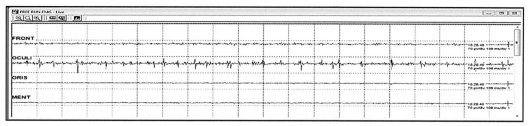

b

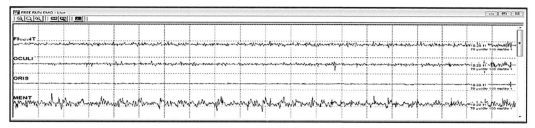

c

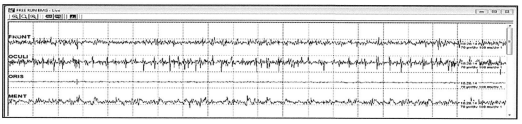

d

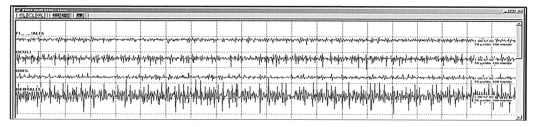

Fig. 5.18 Self free-run EMG activity. EMG is weakly measured only in the oculi (**a**), and EMG is also measured in mentalis (**b**). In this state, if the muscle relaxant is not administered and left as it is, EMG is measured in all facial muscles, and the patient wakes up from anesthesia and moves (**c, d**)

References

1. Park SK, Joo EB, Park K. Intraoperative neurophysiological monitoring during microvascular decompression surgery for hemifacial spasm. J Korean Neurosurg Soc. 2019 Jul;62(4):367–375. https://doi.org/10.3340/jkns.2018.0218. Epub 2019 Jul 1.
2. Sindou M, Mercier P. Microvascular decompression for hemifacial spasm: Surgical techniques and intraoperative monitoring. Neurochirurgie. 2018 May;64(2):133–143. https://doi.org/10.1016/j.neuchi.2018.04.003. Epub 2018 May 18.
3. Prell JRS, Rachinger J, Scheller C, Naraghi R, Strauss C. Spontaneous electromyographic activity during microvascular decompression in trigeminal neuralgia. J Clin Neurophysiol. 2008 Aug;25(4):225–32. https://doi.org/10.1097/WNP.0b013e31817f368f.
4. Romstöck J, Struass C, Fahlbusch R. Continuous electromyography monitoring of motor cranial nerves during cerebellopontine angle surgery. J Neurosurg. 2000 Oct;93(4):586–93. https://doi.org/10.3171/jns.2000.93.4.0586.

5. Kircher ML, Kartush JM. Pitfalls in intraoperative nerve monitoring during vestibular schwannoma surgery. Neurosurg Focus. 2012 Sep;33(3):E5. https://doi.org/10.3171/2012.7.FOCUS12196.

6. Lee S, Park SK, Lee JA, Joo BE, Park K. Missed culprits in failed microvascular decompression surgery for hemifacial spasm and clinical outcomes of redo surgery. World Neurosurg. 2019 Sep;129:e627–e633. https://doi.org/10.1016/j.wneu.2019.05.231. Epub 2019 May 31.

7. Fukuda M, Takao T, Hiraishi T, Fujii Y. Free-running EMG monitoring during microvascular decompression for hemifacial spasm. Acta Neurochir. 2015;157:1505–12.

8. Chung YH, Kim WH, Lee JJ, Yang SI, Lim SH, Seo DW, Park K, Chung IS. Lateral spread response monitoring during microvascular decompression for hemifacial spasm. Anaesthesist. 2014;63:122–128. https://doi.org/10.1007/s00101-013-2286-3. Epub 2014 Feb 7.

6.1 Slowly Extending Latency First, Followed by Amplitude Reduction, Followed by Loss of Waveform (Deafness After Surgery)

The most common pattern in which the BAEPs waveform is lost is that the latency extension of wave V is observed, followed by a decrease in amplitude, and eventually disappears (Fig. 6.1). This change in amplitude after latency change was observed because the degree of damage to the cochlear nerve increased very slowly. In this case, the operation was briefly stopped to recover the BAEPs waveform by interpreting the BAEPs waveform well and giving an appropriate comment to the surgeon. You should be able to do it. Failure to do so will lead to BAEPs loss and eventually lead to patient hearing loss after surgery [1, 2].

The following is the change and explanation of the waveform according to the surgical procedure.

(Fig. 6.1a): Rt. No hearing problems before surgery. Base data (wave V latency 6.5 ms, amplitude 0.2 µV) were measured during surgery in HFS patients

(Fig. 6.1b): After dura open, the cerebellum was retracted using a retractor, the arachnoid membrane was dissected from the rostral of the low cranial nerve, and the area with the choroid plexus was retracted to observe the facial nerve

root exit zone. When the cerebellum was further retraction and exposed to the ventral side, it was observed that the facial nerve was compressed by the AICA. In this dissection of vessel and nerve stage, 1 ms delayed wave V latency was observed, and there was no change in amplitude. In this case, the surgeon must be informed of the wave V latency 1 ms delayed state to recognize that the cochlear nerve is weakly affected. Surgeon was aware of the slight wave extension and continued the operation [1]

(Fig. 6.1c, d): Wave V latency 2 ms delayed was observed during Teflon insertion. However, since the amplitude did not decrease by more than 50%, surgeon quickly and hurriedly performed the surgical operation. Since we know that the change in amplitude is more important than the change in latency, we made this choice [3–5]

(Fig. 6.1e): When the Teflon insertion was completed, the wave V latency was delayed by 2.8 ms, and the amplitude decreased by 50%. Amplitude decreases suddenly within a few seconds, unlike latency extension (Chap. 3, Sect. 3.4). Therefore, in order to sensitively measure the change in amplitude, it is advantageous to test within 10 seconds much faster than the conventional method [6]

(Fig. 6.1f): So I hurriedly removed the brain retractor, but the waveform did not recover but rather disappeared. It can be seen that a delayed wave V latency of 2 ms or more is a very dangerous state as it is considered that the wave V latency is suddenly lost after an extension of 2 ms or more occurs (Chap. 3, Sect. 3.4)

(Fig. 6.1g, h): BAEPs were observed as wave all loss for a while and were thought to have also received vascular circulation damage (Chap. 3, Sects. 3.4 and 3.6). Solumedrol and papaverin were administered to both nerve damage and

blood circulation improvement. I waited for it to get better, but it did not recover

(Fig. 6.1i): After closing the dura, wave I recovered and began to be clearly observed, but the remaining waveforms still did not recover. The presence of wave I in BAEPs wave loss is of great significance. Since cochlear is the origin of the waveform, BAEPs wave loss patients with

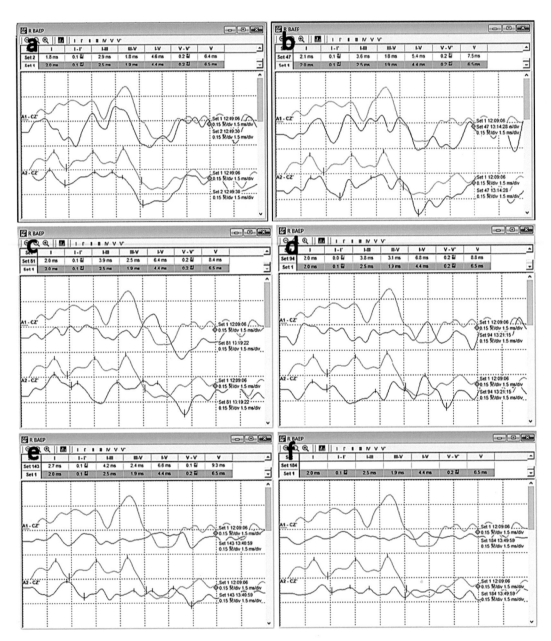

Fig. 6.1 (**a**) Base data; (**b**) dissection of vessel and nerve; (**c**) before Teflon insertion; (**d**) Teflon insertion; (**e**) after Teflon insertion; (**f**) remove brain retractor; (**g, h**) dura closing; (**i**) after dura closed; (**j**) OP closed data

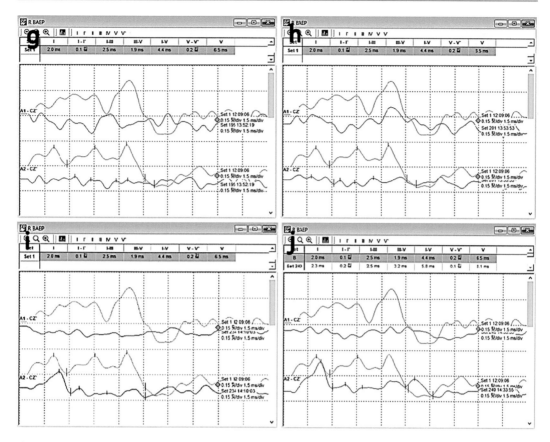

Fig. 6.1 (continued)

wave I only complain of simple deafness symptoms after surgery. However, in case of BAEPs wave all loss without wave I, a problem occurs in the vestibular function as well, resulting in serious dizziness and deafness

(Fig. 6.1j): No waveform was observed except wave I until just before the surgery was completed

After the operation, the patient became totally deaf as a result of the audiometry test. During the operation, wave I was maintained, the remaining waveforms were lost, and the patient's symptoms were consistent with the postoperative symptoms, so there was no dizziness (Fig. 6.2).

If the brain retractor was removed when the wave V latency was delayed by 2 ms during surgery and the BAEPs waveform was restored and then proceeded again, the postoperative deafness would not have occurred. If the operation is continued in the state of 2 ms delayed wave V latency

without amplitude change, amplitude loss occurs, and this condition is a case where the auditory nerve is severely damaged. The function of the cochlear nerve cannot be restored. That is, wave V amplitude, which suddenly decreases by more than 50% within 10 seconds, is a very dangerous warning criterion, but wave V latency 2 ms delayed is also very dangerous.

6.2   Slowly Extending Latency First, Followed by Amplitude Reduction, Followed by Loss of Waveform (Normal After Surgery)

During surgery, BAEPs wave V latency delayed was observed, followed by a decrease in wave V amplitude, and eventually disappeared, showing the same flow as in Chap. 6, Sect. 6.1 (Fig. 6.3).

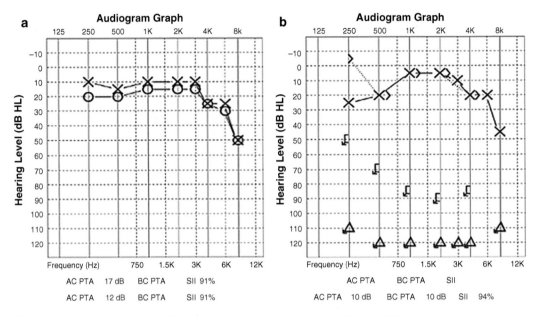

Fig. 6.2 Preoperation pure tone audiometry (**a**), postoperation pure tone audiometry (**b**)

However, this patient gradually recovered and had normal hearing after surgery. In that case, BAEPs loss occurred during surgery, but due to some differences, let's take a closer look at the deafness after surgery in some cases and hearing normal in some cases.

(Fig. 6.3a): Rt. Base data (wave V latency 6.2 ms, amplitude 0.3 μV) were measured during surgery with HFS patients

(Fig. 6.3b): After dura open, the cerebellum was retracted using a retractor, the arachnoid membrane was dissected from the rostral of the low cranial nerve, and the area with the choroid plexus was retracted to observe the facial nerve root exit zone. When the cerebellum was further retraction and exposed to the ventral side, it was observed that the facial nerve was compressed by the AICA. In this situation, if a change in wave V latency occurs due to the influence of the brain retractor, the brain retractor should be released frequently to restore the BAEPs wave to normal. If the wave V amplitude also changes due to the brain retractor, BAEPs loss is likely to occur, so be very careful. Just before the Teflon insertion, a wave V latency of 1 ms delayed was observed, and there was no change in amplitude

(Fig. 6.3c, d): When Teflon insertion was successfully completed, a wave V latency of 2 ms delayed was observed, and a decrease in wave V amplitude was not observed

(Fig. 6.3e, f): In the process of removing the brain retractor and closing the dura, the waveform did not recover, but rather, the wave V latency was delayed by 3.1 ms, and a decrease in the wave V amplitude began to be observed. All waveforms except wave I were lost

(Fig. 6.3g): After the dura was closed, the waveform gradually began to recover, and the wave V latency was delayed by 3.33 ms, and the wave V amplitude decreased by 50%

(Fig. 6.3h): Immediately before the end of the surgery, it was observed that the wave V latency was delayed by 1.5 ms and the wave V amplitude decreased by 20%, and the examination was completed

After surgery, the patient had normal hearing (Fig. 6.4). When analyzing the reason for obtaining these results by the waveform during surgery, surgeon was well aware that the wave V latency was delayed by 1 ms by the brain retractor, and the AICA branch entered the medial side between CN 7 and 8 during the Teflon insertion process. I tried decompressing together, but wave V latency 2 ms delayed was observed, so I think that removing the brain retractor without further proceeding is a very important point. This is because the wave V latency 2 ms delayed state without amplitude change was recognized and prepared for a very dangerous state that could suddenly lead to BAEPs loss (Fig. 6.3e).

In the process of removing the brain retractor and closing the dura, the waveform was not recovered immediately, but rather all the waveforms except wave I were lost. I think that the wave V latency 2 ms delayed state is very dangerous (Fig. 6.3f). Since no more serious damage was inflicted, the waveform gradually began to recover after the dura was closed, and the influence on the floccules by the retractor during Teflon insertion was not completely recovered, so the waveform recovered 80% of the wave V amplitude at the end of the surgery, and wave V latency is still significantly extended to 3.33 ms (Fig. 6.3h) (Chap. 3, Sects. 3.3, and 3.6).

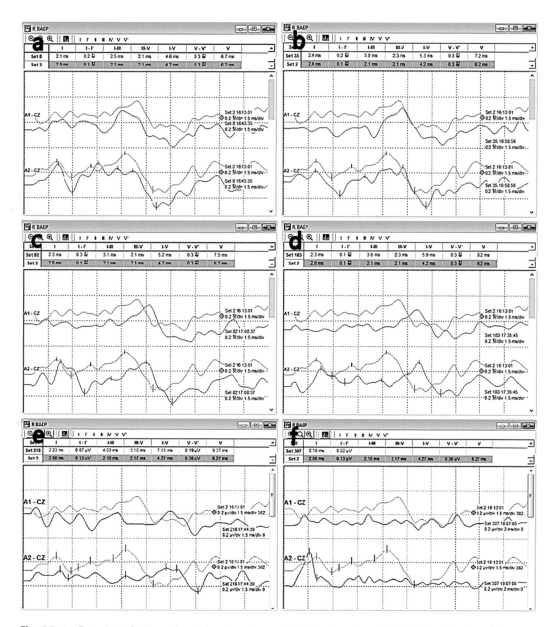

Fig. 6.3 (**a**) Base data; (**b**) dissection of vessel and nerve; (**c**) Teflon insertion; (**d**) after Teflon insertion; (**e**) remove brain retractor; (**f**) dura closing; (**g**) after dura closed; (**h**) OP closed data

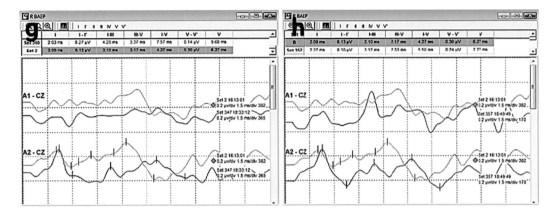

Fig. 6.3 (continued)

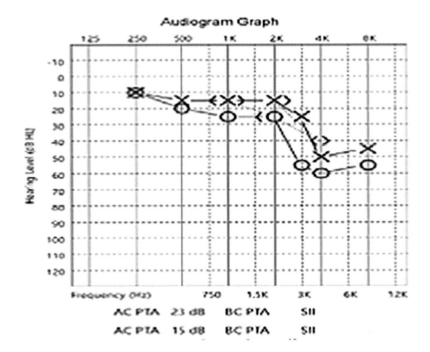

Fig. 6.4 Pre-/postoperation pure tone audiometry remains unchanged

Postoperative PTA results were normal for patients as before surgery. BAEPs In the case where wave loss occurs and the body surgery for which the waveform has not been recovered is terminated, the patient's condition after surgery varies greatly depending on the presence of wave I.

- First, when the operation is terminated due to BAEPs wave loss while wave I is present, more than 50% of patients show normal hearing after surgery. This is thought to be because the damaged cochlear nerve recovers very slowly. In other words, it is thought that the operation was ended in a state in which the waveform lost during the operation could not be recovered. And deafness occurs in the rest of the patients. The reason for this is that the cochlear nerve was severely affected so that it was not possible to recover. It is difficult to determine the degree of damage to the cochlear nerve in the case where the surgery is terminated due to wave loss of BAEPs with wave I present. What is only certain is that if the wave is recovered after BAEPs wave loss during surgery, the postoperative hearing is normal.

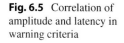

Fig. 6.5 Correlation of amplitude and latency in warning criteria

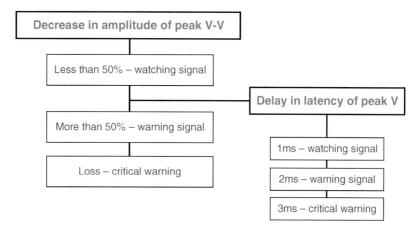

- Second, if the operation is terminated with BAEPs wave all loss where wave I does not exist, 100% deafness occurs after surgery. The problem with vascular circulation has caused problems for the cochlear itself. Therefore, since even wave I is also lost, it is affected by the vestibular function, and dizziness is accompanied [7].

So, we set the new BAEPs warning criteria for BAEPs wave V amplitude and latency. It was presented in 3.2 and is as follows (Fig. 6.5), and it is recommended to take measures to recover the BAEPs wave when the wave V amplitude and latency correspond to the warning signal.

Warning criteria applied when using real-time BAEPs. The relationship between latency and amplitude is presented separately based on wave V. In real-time BAEPs tests, latency changes were always observed first, followed by amplitude changes. In addition, latency change was observed slowly and continuously, and amplitude change suddenly decreased by more than 50% within 10 seconds.

6.3   When the Amplitude Suddenly Decreases and the Waveform Disappears Without Extending Latency (Deafness After Surgery)

In general, the change in the BAEPs wave is observed to be prolonged in the wave V latency, and the pattern in which the amplitude decreases

after that is because the damage to the cochlear nerve proceeds very weakly and gradually. Wave V latency is often extended to less than 1 ms simply by dura open. In other words, even with a very weak influence, the wave V latency may change. And when we see that the amplitude changes after the change in wave V latency is always observed, it can be seen that the change in amplitude is changed by a more serious influence than the latency. Therefore, when BAEPs wave change suddenly changes in amplitude without change in latency, it is because the cochlear nerve was severely damaged in a short time without weak effects such as stretching of the cochlear nerve.

If the brain retractor is suddenly and severely affected, the wave V amplitude suddenly decreases by more than 50% without changing the wave V latency (Fig. 6.6). In the case of more severe influence, only wave I exists, and all other waveforms are lost. And in order to discriminate from such a sudden and serious impact, it is much easier to perform the test in less than 10 seconds [6]. If a waveform is observed in progressive form, such as when the wave V latency extension is observed and then the amplitude of the amplate is also reduced and the waveform is lost, the waveform's observation can be quickly addressed when the waveform is lost because it is aware of the waveform change even before the waveform is lost.

In other words, if the retractor is frequently removed so that the waveform can be recovered before the wave V latency 2 ms delayed, the decrease in amplitude can be prevented. However,

Fig. 6.6 Waveform loss
after sudden wave V
amplitude decrease

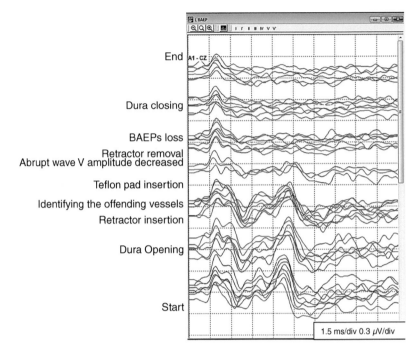

if the amplitude suddenly decreases or disappears by more than 50% without changing the wave V latency, it is difficult to cope with it quickly, and the reduced waveform does not recover well. This is thought to be due to severe focal mechanical damage, and this phenomenon is very dangerous because it causes deafness after surgery. The characteristic point is that wave I always exists and all other waveforms are lost. After surgery, low-frequency hearing loss occurs in most cases (Fig. 6.7), and total-frequency hearing loss occurs if very seriously affected.

6.4   When There Is No Change in Latency and Amplitude During the Main Procedure, and the Waveform Disappears After Closing the Dura (Deafness After Surgery)

(Fig. 6.8a): Rt. Base data (wave V latency 6.3 ms, amplitude 0.35 µV) were measured during surgery in HFS patients

(Fig. 6.8b, c): No change in waveform was observed until after dura open

(Fig. 6.8d, e): At the stage of dissection of vessels and nerves and identifying the offending ves-

sels, wave V latency of 0.67 ms delayed was observed without a change in amplitude

(Fig. 6.8f, g): Teflon pad insertion was made between CN 7 and CN 8 as the offending site, and when the brain retractor was removed, it was observed that the latency was recovering with a wave V latency of 0.37 ms delayed

(Fig. 6.8h): After the dura was closed, all the BAEPs waveforms were lost without wave I, so when the dura was opened again, AICA vasospasm was observed. So, papaverine was administered but the waveform did not recover. This is a phenomenon that occurred 13 minutes after removing the brain retractor. This delayed BAEPs loss phenomenon is very rare. If the BAEPs change caused by vasospasm is detected and responded more quickly, the lost waveform may be recovered (Fig. 6.10). Therefore, it is important to observe the waveform change by performing the BAEPs test until the operation is completed

(Fig. 6.8i): The surgery for the body without recovering the lost waveform was completed

The patient had no facial spasms after the operation but complained of tinnitus, hearing loss, and loss of balance (Fig. 6.9). In the case of BAEPs all loss where even wave I is not observed when BAEPs loss occurs, complica-

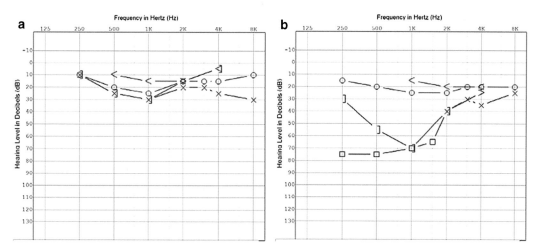

Fig. 6.7 Preoperation pure tone audiometry (**a**), postoperation pure tone audiometry (**b**)

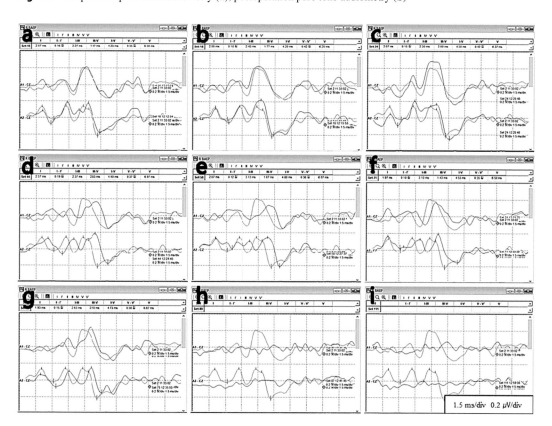

Fig. 6.8 (**a**) Base data; (**b**) before dura open; (**c**) after dura open; (**d**) dissection of vessel and nerve; (**e**) identifying the offending vessels; (**f**) Teflon pad insertion; (**g**) dura closing; (**h**) after dura closed; (**i**) OP closed data

tions such as tinnitus, dizziness, diplopia, and hoarseness are additionally generated in addition to deafness [7].

6.5 Conclusion

When BAEPs wave V latency is gradually delayed during surgery and then the amplitude

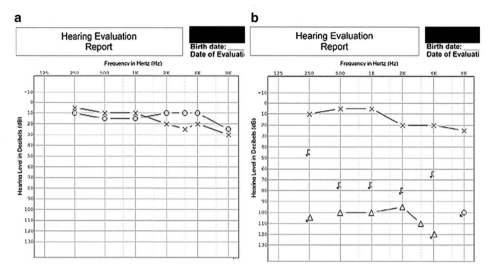

Fig. 6.9 Preoperation pure tone audiometry (**a**), postoperation pure tone audiometry (**b**)

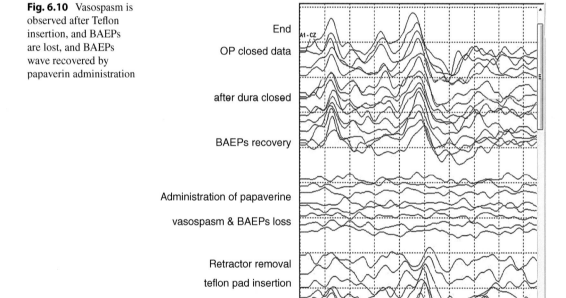

Fig. 6.10 Vasospasm is observed after Teflon insertion, and BAEPs are lost, and BAEPs wave recovered by papaverin administration

decreases by 50%, it is mostly caused by the influence of the brain retractor. In this case, when the brain retractor is removed, the waveform is recovered very well. However, the sudden decrease in amplitude by 50% without change in

BAEPs wave V latency is a much more dangerous condition than gradually showing a change in latency and leading to a decrease in amplitude by 50%. When the amplitude suddenly decreases by 50%, remove the brain retractor, and if you do not wait for this to recover, it can lead to BAEPs loss, so be careful.

During surgery, a stable waveform was observed without changes in BAEPs, or BAEPs change occurred several times, and even if recovery was performed, BAEPs loss may occur by the time the dura is closed. Therefore, BAEPs should be tested until the operation is completed. This is because BAEPs all loss without wave I is mostly due to a problem in the blood circulation of the labyrinthine artery, which supplies blood to the vestibular cochlear nerve. Therefore, when the surgery is terminated due to BAEPs all loss without wave I, complications accompanied by dizziness as well as HL after surgery occur.

References

1. Park SK, Joo BE, Lee S, Lee JA, Hwang JH, Kong DS, Seo DW, Park K, Lee HT. The critical warning sign of real-time brainstem auditory evoked potentials during microvascular decompression for hemifacial spasm. Clin Neurophysiol. 2018 May;129(5):1097–1102. https://doi.org/10.1016/j.clinph.2017.12.032. Epub 2018 Jan 4.
2. Thirumala PD, Carnovale G, Habeych ME, Crammond DJ, Balzer JR. Diagnostic accuracy of brainstem auditory evoked potentials during microvascular decompression. Neurology. 2014 Nov 4;83(19):1747–1752. https://doi.org/10.1212/WNL.0000000000000961. Epub 2014 Oct 8.
3. Legatt AD. Mechanisms of intraoperative brainstem auditory evoked potential changes. J Clin Neurophysiol. 2002 Oct;19(5):396–408. https://doi.org/10.1097/00004691-200210000-00003.
4. Jo KW, Kim JW, Kong DS, Hong SH, Park K. The patterns and risk factors of hearing loss following microvascular decompression for hemifacial spasm. Acta Neurochir (Wien). 2011 May;153(5):1023–1030. https://doi.org/10.1007/s00701-010-0935-8. Epub 2011 Jan 15.
5. Jung NY, Lee SW, Park CK, Chang WS, Jung HH, Chang JW. Hearing outcome following microvascular decompression for hemifacial spasm: series of 1434 cases. World Neurosurg. 2017 Dec;108:566–571. https://doi.org/10.1016/j.wneu.2017.09.053. Epub 2017 Sep 18.
6. Joo BE, Park SK, Cho KR, Kong DS, Seo DW, Park K. Real-time intraoperative monitoring of brainstem auditory evoked potentials during microvascular decompression for hemifacial spasm. J Neurosurg. 2016;125:1061–1067. https://doi.org/10.3171/2015.10.JNS151224. Epub 2016 Jan 29.
7. Joo BE, Park SK, Lee MH, Lee S, Lee JA, Park K. Significance of wave I loss of brainstem auditory evoked potentials during microvascular decompression surgery for hemifacial spasm. Clin Neurophysiol. 2020 Apr;131(4):809–815. https://doi.org/10.1016/j.clinph.2019.12.409. Epub 2020 Jan 21.

Artifacts of Intraoperative Neurophysiological Monitoring

7.1 Artifacts

7.1.1 Electrical Artifact

7.1.1.1 Electrical Artifact (Electrical Power)

A variety of different machines can be found in the operating room. The NIOM team must know not only their function but also the effect they can have on monitoring. Many machines will produce high-amplitude artifacts that must be recognized. In detail, there are studies that reported that electrocautery, microscope and monitor, cavitron ultrasonic surgical aspirator (CUSA), and surgical table are applicable [1, 2].

Among the evoked potential waveforms, the smallest potential is the BAEPs waveform. Motor evoked potentials (MEP), visual evoked potentials (VEP), somatosensory evoked potentials (SEP), and free-running EMG are amplitudes ranging from 2 µV to 1 mV. Within the range, 60 Hz wave artifacts are mixed into the waveform [3]. However, the BAEPs waveform itself has an amplitude of 0.2 µV to 0.3 µV, which is too small with an amplitude of 1/10 compared to other waveforms, so when electrical artifacts are mixed, the waveform itself cannot be distinguished (Fig. 7.1). Therefore, the electrical power of the test equipment must be grounded with stable medical power to prevent electrical artifacts from being mixed.

Generally, hospital grade electrical facilities are installed in hospitals. Standards such as NEMA-6 (National Electrical Manufacturers Association), which is a medical power standard in the United States, is suitable for testing all evoked potentials as well as BAEPs because the voltage fluctuation is small, and the grounding is very stable (Figs. 7.2 and 7.3). If the equipment power cable is connected to the same place as the extension cable, it cannot be ruled out that the main power source of the extension cable is plugged into a place other than medical power, and if the equipment does not have adequate socket–outlets to be used, it may not be possible to inspect the BAEPs themselves due to the mixture of electrical effects, so be very careful.

Even if the electrical power of the test equipment is plugged into a medical power whose ground is stable, care should be taken because the grounding function does not work smoothly even if it is slightly pushed out of the wall, and noise may occur in the test waveform (Fig. 7.4).

7.1.1.2 Electrical Artifact (Operation Bed)

The surgical bed used in neurosurgery is a bed that adjusts the height and moves using electricity. Because it is designed to charge electricity, the bed works without plugging in the outlet for a certain period of time. However, when the bed is used for a long time, there are often cases of problems with charging. As the charged electricity

S.-K. Park et al., *Intraoperative Neurophysiological Monitoring in Hemifacial Spasm*, https://doi.org/10.1007/978-981-16-1327-2_7

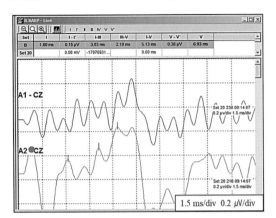

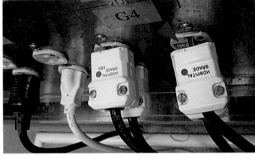

Fig. 7.4 Power cable slightly protruding from the wall

Fig. 7.1 BAEPs waveform with electrical artifacts

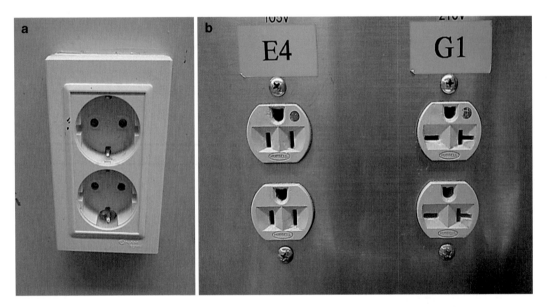

Fig. 7.2 General power outlet (**a**) and medical power outlet (**b**)

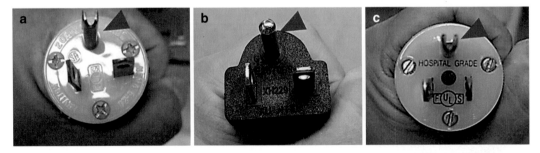

Fig. 7.3 The power cable for medical power is designed to strengthen the ground function, so it can prevent the mixing of electrical artifacts as much as possible. 220 V medical power plug assembly type (**a**), 220 V medical power plug integral type (**b**), 110 V medical power plug assembly type (**c**)

becomes very weak and little by little electric leakage, there is a case that it affects minute waveforms such as BAEPs. In this case, it is observed that electrical noise is mixed enough to affect the free-running EMG, and the LSR test may be difficult to judge [4]. In the situation where such artifacts occur, a stable waveform can be implemented because the micro-current that caused electric leakage is resolved by the grounding of the medical power when the bed power cord is plugged in.

There is also the opposite phenomenon. When the bed power cord is well plugged in, there are cases where artifacts are seriously mixed in the waveform of BAEPs. In this case, the grounding function in the power cable itself is a faulty cable. There is no problem with the supply of medical power to the bed, but the electricity remaining after use in the bed must be safely recovered. If there is a problem with the grounding function, the electric leakage is caused by electric leakage. In this case, it can be solved by unplugging the

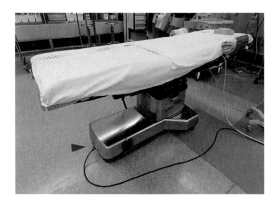

Fig. 7.5 Operation bed

bed power cord or replacing it with another new one (Fig. 7.5).

All medical devices related to surgery that use electricity, as well as the surgical bed, fall under these conditions, so you should be familiar with them.

It is the surgical bed that has the most artifacts on the examination during surgery. Connecting or disconnecting the power cable can solve the electrical artifacts caused by the bed.

7.1.2 Head Fixator Artifact

The patient's head is fixed with a headrest or a head holder, and surgery is performed, but there is a peculiar artifact that occurs only when the head is fixed with a head holder.

In MVD surgery, one pin is fixed on the forehead on the side of the surgery area, and the other two are fixed on the back of the head (Fig. 7.6). The head is opened when completely fixed. Open the skull suitable for surgery, and after dura open, perform the surgery by retraction so that the surgical site is clearly visible using a spatula (brain retractor). Unusually, the BAEPs waveform, which was smoothly measured at the beginning of the surgery, sometimes generates artifacts only while manipulating the brain retractor, making it impossible to determine the waveform at all.

The reason that it can be concluded that it is the effect of the brain retractor is that it occurs only when the brain retractor is manipulated, and BAEPs occur as artifacts are generated in the frontalis of the pin area and the free-running EMG of the oculi fixed on the forehead of the surgical site. This is because waveforms cannot

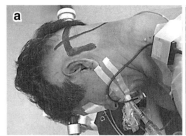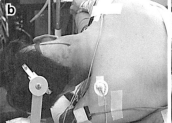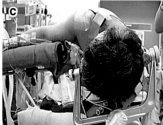

Fig. 7.6 Head holder and fixation, side view (**a**), back view (**b**), top view (**c**)

be measured. Artifact is characterized by the fact that the free-running EMG of the frontalis and the oculi is symmetrical to each other in the same shape as a bridge wave (Fig. 7.7).

When using the brain retractor, it is used for the main procedure, and BAEPs waveform should be monitored most intensively, but it becomes very difficult if BAEPs waveform measurement is not possible due to unknown effects.

This phenomenon is similarly observed when using a bone drill (Fig. 7.8), and in the case of fixing the head using a head holder, the EEG wave or VEP wave is also caused by artifacts for the same reason whenever the brain retractor is moved. An obstacle occurs in the formation of the waveform (Fig. 7.9).

Even while opening the bones of the head with a drill, the shape of the artifact is only mixed

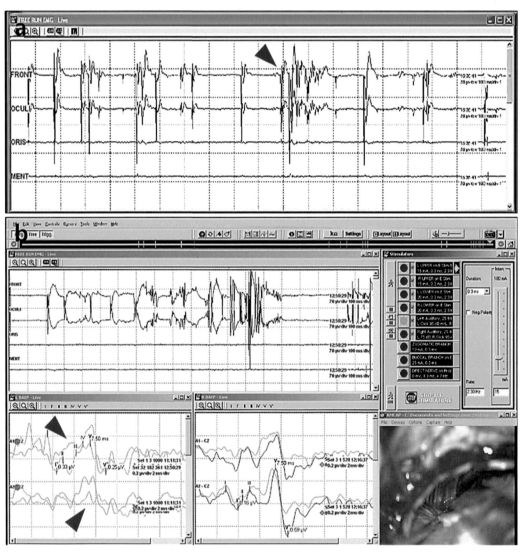

Fig. 7.7 Brain retractor artifact. It is characteristic that the frontalis and oculi free-running EMG are symmetrical to each other in the same shape as a bridge wave (**a**), and

in this case, it affects the BAEPs waveform and causes a big problem that the waveform cannot be formed (**b**)

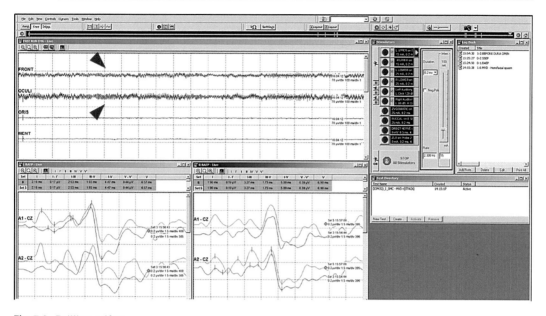

Fig. 7.8 Drilling artifact

with the free-running EMG of the frontalis and oculi.

There is a way to solve this problem. Looking at the cause of these artifacts, it is judged that it occurs only when the brain retractor is moved, so that it occurs at the joints of the primary bar, secondary bar, and arm retractor. This artifact can be completely removed by applying dry gauze at the first area where the head holder and primary bar meet, as it does not affect the EMG (Fig. 7.10).

And even if the brain retractor and muscle retractor are attached to each other, noise is generated, which may interfere with the BAEPs test. Therefore, even if the brain retractor is not used, it must be separated from the muscle retractor (Fig. 7.11).

7.1.3 Microscope Artifact

After the operation started, the BAEPs were examined and the base data was well measured. When the microscope is pulled close to the patient's bed to see the microscope, the BAEPs waveform suddenly generates noise, and the examination may not be smooth. In this case, it is because the distance between the microscope and the BAEPs's measuring electrode is too close, so

it can be solved by removing the microscope from the patient's head a little apart. However, moving the microscope back and forth while the BAEPs waveform is abruptly not measured during surgery may interfere with the operation, so this problem can be solved by consulting a surgeon in advance to determine an appropriate distance to move the microscope to be used.

It is easy to secure a stable distance between the microscope and the bed when the position of the operation bed is fixed in advance (Fig. 7.12).

7.1.4 Facial Nerve EMG Artifact

When a Teflon pad is inserted between the offending vessel and the facial nerve, a free-running EMG waveform naturally occurs. However, whenever the free-running EMG waveform is measured, the BAEPs waveform may not be measured smoothly (Fig. 7.13). In general, the auricular area used as the A1 or A2 position in the BAEPs test is difficult to use because it is close to the surgical site (Fig. 7.14a).

So, the places used for other parts are shown in Fig. 7.14b, c site. In this area, the position A1 or A2, which is used as a measuring electrode for BAEPs, corresponds to the peripheral distal

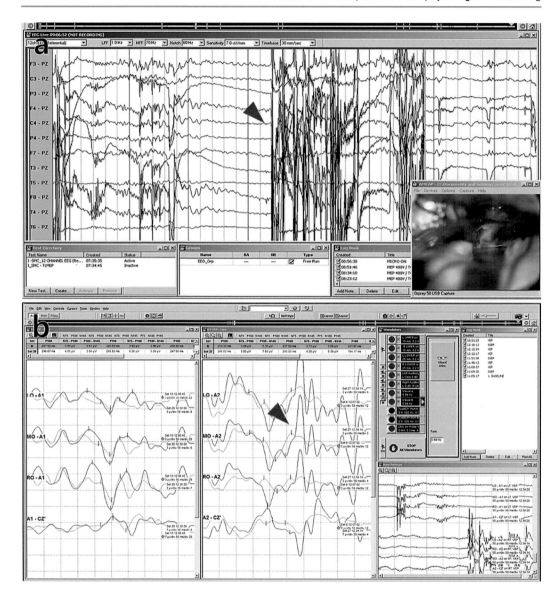

Fig. 7.9 Even in EEG (**a**) and VEP (**b**) tests, artifacts are generated equally each time the brain retractor is moved, affecting the waveform

branch of the facial nerve, so every time the facial nerve is touched by surgical manipulation, a free-running EMG waveform is generated, and thereby A1 or A2 is affected. As a result, the BAEPs waveform is not smooth.

This happens very rarely, but it is a phenomenon that should never occur during surgery to preserve the patient's hearing by allowing smooth BAEPs to be measured. To prevent such artifacts

from occurring, it may be a good idea to select the A1 or A2 position used as the BAEPs's measuring electrode as tragus or antitragus. If the tubal insert phone is inserted into the ear hole, the subdermal needle electrode is inserted right next to it, and the auricle is folded and fixed; it is not affected by the free-running EMG waveform caused by surgical manipulation of the facial nerve, and the fixation is safe, so it is very effective (Fig. 7.14)

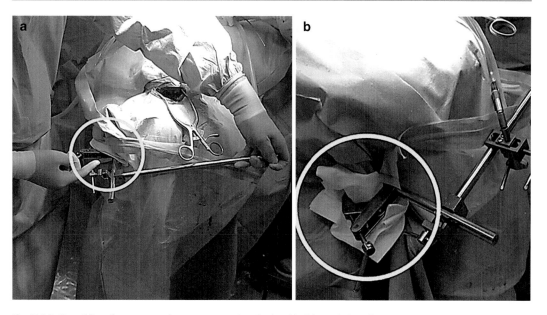

Fig. 7.10 By adding dry gauze to the area connecting the head holder and the primary bar, the influence of the movement of the brain retractor can be blocked

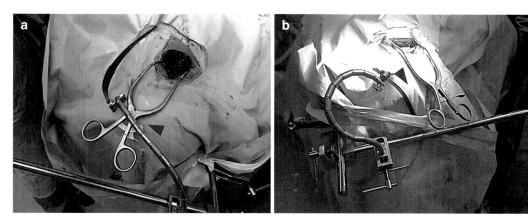

Fig. 7.11 Even if the brain retractor and muscle retractor are attached to each other, noise is generated, which interferes with the BAEPs test (**a**). Therefore, even if the brain retractor is not used, it must be separated from the muscle retractor (**b**)

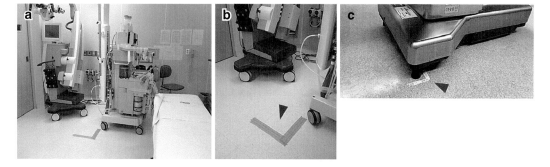

Fig. 7.12 Make and mark the boundary of the distance that the microscope can approach to the bed (**a, b**), and mark the location so that the location of the operation bed is always at the same location (**c**)

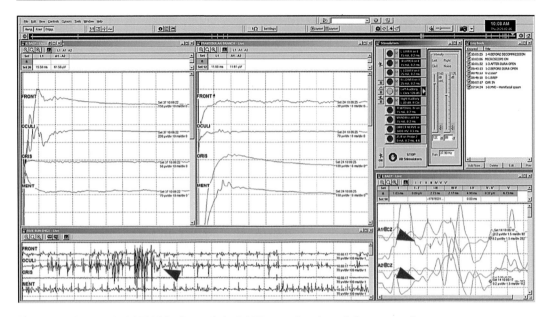

Fig. 7.13 Whenever facial EMG is observed, the BAEPs waveform is not being measured

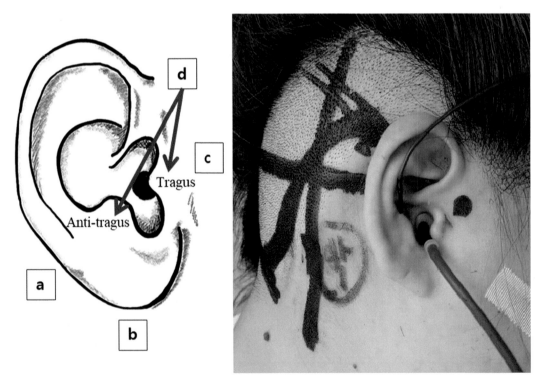

Fig. 7.14 Photographs of electrodes inserted on the tragus, anti-tragus. The facial nerve can only be touched by manipulation during surgery. In this case, if the BAEPs electrode is installed in the facial nerve peripheral branch, it can be affected and not measured smoothly

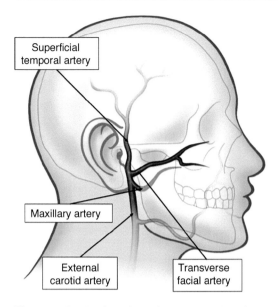

Fig. 7.15 On the front face of the tragus, there is an external carotid artery, a transverse facial artery and a maxillary artery branching there, and a superficial temporal artery origin

Figure 7.14a and b are not used because there is a risk of contamination because they are too close to the area to be operated on, and it is covered with dressing gauze at the surgical site even after the needle electrode is removed after surgery, so it is difficult to determine the infection state of the electrode removal site.

Figure 7.14c Inserting an electrode in the area can affect the BAEPs waveform when touching the facial nerve, as well as the external carotid artery on the front face of the tragus and the transverse facial artery and maxillary artery branching there, removing the electrode. After bleeding may occur seriously, so be very careful (Fig. 7.15)

References

1. Lee GRI. Book review: A practical approach to neurophysiologic intraoperative monitoring, 2nd Edition. J Clin Neurophysiol. 2016 Oct;33(5):476.
2. Nuwer MR. Regulatory and medical-legal aspects of intraoperative monitoring. J Clin Neurophysiol. 2002 Oct;19(5):387–95.
3. Shirai Y. Special characteristics and necessary equipments for intraoperative neurological monitoring. Rinsho Byori. 2008 Jun;56(6):465–74.
4. Urriza J, Ulkatan S, Deletis V. Shuffle the puzzle: Spinal motor-evoked potentials vs. 50-Hz artifact. Asian Cardiovasc Thorac Ann. 2015 Jul;23(6):754–5.

BAEPs Wave and Hearing Loss

8.1 Relationship Between Hearing Loss Patients and BAEPs Waveform

Is there a case where the BAEPs waveform is normal when the patient has poor hearing? (Fig. 8.1)

The ear consists of three parts: the outer ear, the middle ear, and the inner ear.

The outer ear consists of the ear canal extending from the head to the ear canal and eardrum.

The middle ear consists of the eardrum, ossicles, and ear canals. The eardrum is a thin membrane that transmits the vibrations of sound transmitted from the ear canal to the ossicles. The ossicles transmit the vibrations of sound transmitted to the eardrum to the inner ear. In addition, the middle ear is connected to the pharynx via the transfer tube. The ear canal maintains the balance of air pressure inside and outside the eardrum by controlling the air in and out.

The inner ear in the skull consists of the cochlea, the triangular duct (semiring bone duct), and the vestibule. The cochlea has hair cells that sense sound transmitted by vibrations from the ossicles. Semicircular canal consists of three semiring-shaped pipes and balances the body with the vestibule.

If you can't hear sound well, it's because there's a problem somewhere in the process of passing the sound through the ears, through the cochlea and nerves, and into the brain. The cause of the problem is very diverse, but depending on where the problem is in the process of recognizing external sound, it is largely divided into conductive hearing loss and sensory neural hearing loss.

• Conductive Hearing Loss

Problems in the ear canal during the transmission of sound are called conductive hearing loss. The causes of conductive hearing loss are very diverse, including inflammation of the ear canal or blockage caused by earwax, damage to the eardrum, otitis media exudative, chronic otitis media, and malfunction of the inner ear bone.

In the case of conductive hearing loss, it is not impossible to hear the sound, but it is less audible than the other side. This occurs due to a structural problem, and since the sound stimulus is slightly delayed to the auditory nerve and transmitted, the BAEPs wave induced by the auditory nerve may have decreased amplitude or delayed latency.

• Sensory Neural Hearing Loss

If the vibrations of sound are well transmitted to the cochlea, the cochlea converts these vibrations into nerve signals using sensory nerve cells

Fig. 8.1 The structure of the ear and BAEPs wave formations. External ear (**a**), middle ear (**b**), inner ear (**c**), conductive hearing loss (**d**), sensory neural hearing loss (**e**). The region from which BAEPs waves I, III, and V are derived (blue arrows). (Color figure online)

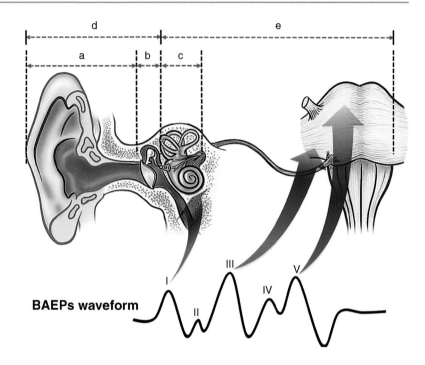

and transmits them to the brain through nerves. If there is a problem in this process, it is called sensorineural hearing loss or neurogenic hearing loss. The causes of sensorineural hearing loss are congenital hearing loss, which is a problem in the neurotransmitting process of sound from birth, noise-induced hearing loss in which nerve cells are damaged by strong noise, sudden hearing loss in which the hearing is suddenly greatly reduced without knowing the cause, and the hearing gradually decreases. Hearing loss may occur due to complications from senile hearing loss, drug toxicity due to drugs that destroy cochlear nerve cells, Meniere's disease, or chronic otitis media.

Sensorineural hearing loss is classified as partial hearing loss in the audible frequency band, in which a specific area is not heard, and is classified into low-frequency hearing loss, high-frequency hearing loss, and mild hearing loss.

Even if you cannot hear a specific frequency due to sensorineural hearing loss, the sound transmission path is structurally normal, and the acoustic nerve is generally excited by sound

stimulation, so the BAEPs wave induced by the auditory nerve can be measured as normal.

- Classification of Hearing Loss

To define HL, we conduct pure tone audiometry (PTA) and speech discrimination scoring (SDS). PTA and SDS are performed on all patients prior to surgery, and both tests are repeated 7 days after surgery. The average PTA thresholds for 500, 1000, 2000, and 4000 Hz were calculated. We determined postoperative HL status by using the most reliable Association of Otolaryngology-Head and Neck Society (AAO-HNS) classification system (1995).

Postoperative HL (class C/D) was defined as PTA > 50 dB and/or SDS < 50% within the speech frequency range.

During preoperative hearing evaluations, patients with preoperative HL (classes C and D) were excluded from the analysis.

Patients with postoperative HL were classified depending on the frequency of PTA indicating HL as follows: low-frequency HL, high-frequency HL, and total-frequency HL.

Low-frequency HL was defined as PTA > 50 dB at 500 and 1000 Hz; high-frequency HL was defined as PTA > 50 dB at 2000 and 4000 Hz. Total-frequency HL was defined as PTA > 50 dB at all measured frequencies [1, 2].

8.1.1 Conductive Hearing Loss

8.1.1.1 Left-Side Conductive Hearing Loss Patient

Rt. HFS F/56 patient who had left conductive hearing loss before surgery (Fig. 8.2a). In the pre-operative BAEPs test, there was no difference in

wave V latency, and the amplitude was 0.19 μV on the left and 0.22 μV on the right.

During the surgery, there was no difference in wave V latency in the BAEPs waveform, and the amplitude was 0.33 μV on the left and 0.35 μV on the right, which was slightly smaller in the area with hearing loss (Fig. 8.2c).

8.1.1.2 Right-Side Conductive Hearing Loss Patient

Lt. HFS M/55 patient who had right conductive hearing loss before surgery (Fig. 8.3a). The waveform of the BAEPs test before surgery was similar to the left and right sides (Fig. 8.3b).

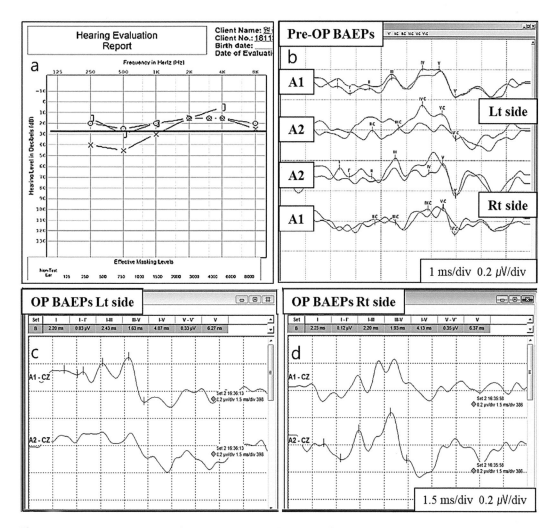

Fig. 8.2 Preoperative pure tone audiometry (**a**), preoperative BAEPs (**b**), intraoperative BAEPs (**c**, **d**)

During surgery, there was no difference in wave V latency in the BAEPs waveform, and the amplitude was 0.35 μV on the left and 0.27 μV on the right, which was slightly smaller in the area with hearing loss (Fig. 8.3c, d).

8.1.1.3 Left-Side Conductive Hearing Loss Patient

Lt. HFS F/48 patient, who had left conductive hearing loss before surgery (Fig. 8.4a). As for the preoperative BAEPs test waveform, a waveform with an extended left wave V latency of 0.3 ms was observed (Fig. 8.4b).

There was no difference in wave V amplitude in the BAEPs during surgery, and the latency was 6.63 ms on the left and 6.53 ms on the right.

8.1.1.4 Right-Side Conductive Hearing Loss Patient

Rt. HFS M/57 patient who had right conductive hearing loss before surgery (Fig. 8.5a). In the preoperative BAEPs test, the wave V latency of the area with the right hearing loss was extended by 0.52 ms, and the amplitude was measured to be slightly smaller than 0.01 μV (Fig. 8.5b).

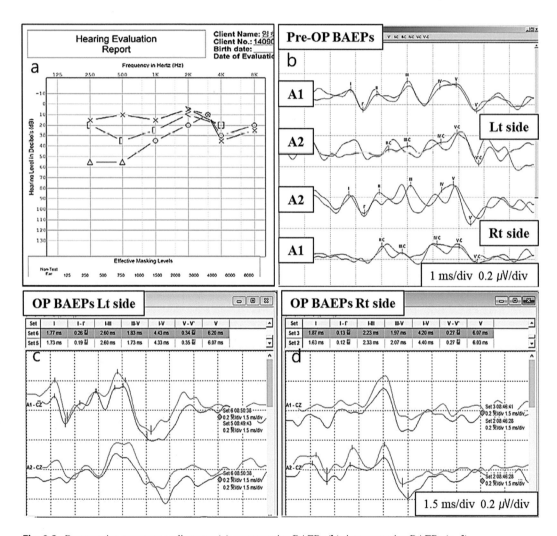

Fig. 8.3 Preoperative pure tone audiometry (**a**), preoperative BAEPs (**b**), intraoperative BAEPs (**c, d**)

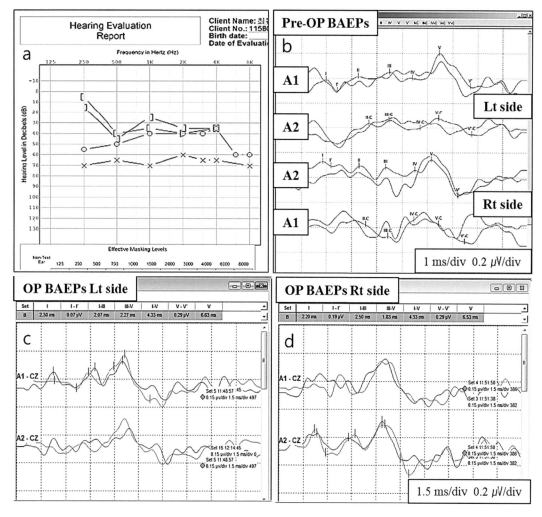

Fig. 8.4 Preoperative pure tone audiometry (**a**), preoperative BAEPs (**b**), intraoperative BAEPs (**c**, **d**)

In the BAEPs during surgery, the wave V latency of the area with the right hearing loss was extended by 1.2 ms, and the amplitude was measured similarly to the left and right (Fig. 8.5c).

8.1.2   Conclusion

Comprehensively, the relationship between conductive hearing loss and BAEPs waves showed that a slight decrease in wave V amplitude was observed in the case of hearing loss in the low-frequency region and hearing loss that can be heard from 50 to 80 dB in the high-frequency region. In the case of, a delay of wave V latency was observed (Table 8.1). This is because the sound transmission is delayed in the ear canal. In particular, since the sound stimulation frequency of the test equipment is 1 KHz, it is thought that the waveform is affected by high-frequency hearing loss.

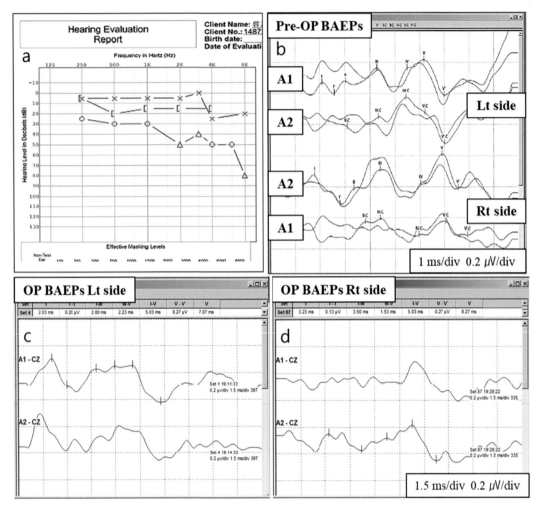

Fig. 8.5 Preoperative pure tone audiometry (**a**), preoperative BAEPs (**b**), intraoperative BAEPs (**c, d**)

Table 8.1 Relationship between conducted hearing loss and BAEPs wave

Conductive hearing loss	BAEPs wave
250–1000 Hz HL	Wave V amplitude 0.02 μV decreased
250–2000 Hz HL	Wave V amplitude 0.08 μV decreased
250–8000 Hz HL	Wave V latency 0.1 ms delayed
2000–8000 Hz HL	Wave V latency 1.2 ms delayed

8.1.3 Sensory Neural Hearing Loss

8.1.3.1 Both-Side High-Frequency Sensory Neural Hearing Loss Patient

Rt. HFS F/47 patient, who had weak bilateral high-frequency hearing loss before surgery (Fig. 8.6a). There was no difference in left and right in the preoperative BAEPs test

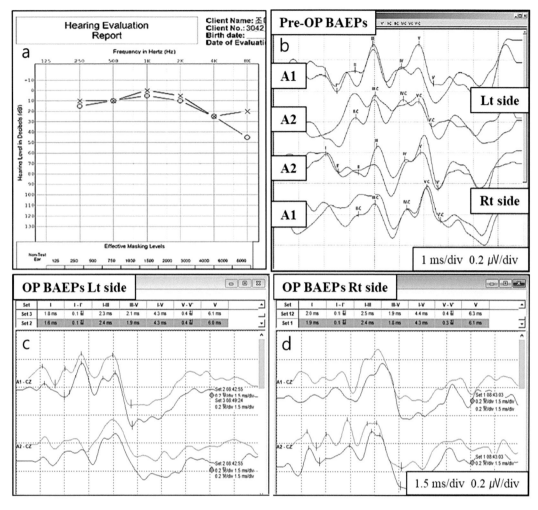

Fig. 8.6 Pure tone audiometry before surgery (**a**), BAEPs before surgery (**b**), BAEPs during surgery (**c, d**)

(Fig. 8.6b), and there was no difference in left and right in the BAEPs waveform during surgery (Fig. 8.6c).

8.1.3.2 Both-Side High-Frequency Sensory Neural Hearing Loss Patient

Lt. HFS F/66 patient who had moderate bilateral high-frequency hearing loss before surgery (Fig. 8.7a). There was no difference between left and right in the preoperative BAEPs test (Fig. 8.7b), and there was no difference between left and right in the BAEPs waveform during surgery (Fig. 8.7c).

8.1.3.3 Both-Side High-Frequency Sensory Neural Hearing Loss Patient

Rt. HFS M/71 patient with severe bilateral high-frequency hearing loss before surgery and a little more severe left side (Fig. 8.8a). There was no difference between left and right in BAEPs waveform during surgery (Fig. 8.8b, c).

8.1.3.4 Both-Side High-Frequency Sensory Neural Hearing Loss Patient

Rt. HFS F/71 patient with severe bilateral high-frequency hearing loss before surgery and a little

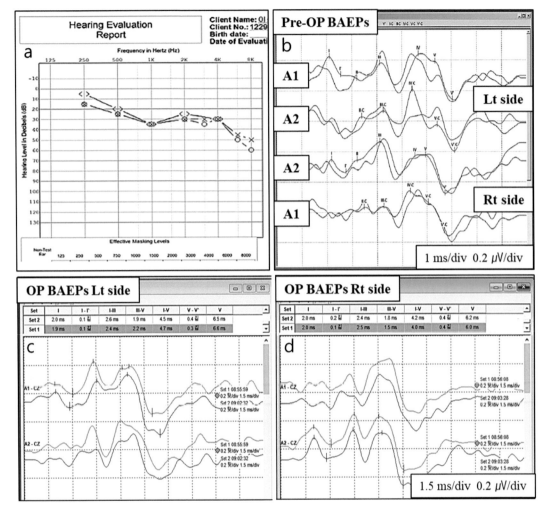

Fig. 8.7 Preoperative pure tone audiometry (**a**), preoperative BAEPs (**b**), intraoperative BAEPs (**c**, **d**)

more severe right side (Fig. 8.9a). There was no difference between left and right in BAEPs waveform during surgery (Fig. 8.9b).

8.1.3.5 Left-Side Total Hearing Loss Patient

Rt. HFS M/64 patient, left deaf before surgery (Fig. 8.10a). During the surgery, the left waveform was not formed in the BAEPs waveform (Fig. 8.10b).

8.1.4 Conclusion

Comprehensively, the relationship between sensory neural hearing loss and BAEPs wave showed that the BAEPs waveform was measured as well as the other side without hearing loss, even though the hearing loss was severe enough to be able to hear even at around 70 dB.

The reason for this is that the sound transmission path is structurally normal even in the case of

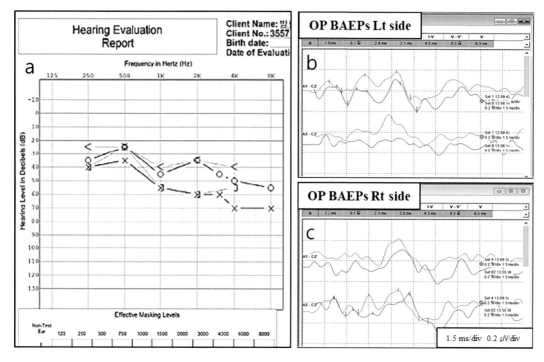

Fig. 8.8 Preoperative pure tone audiometry (**a**), preoperative BAEPs (**b**), intraoperative BAEPs (**c**)

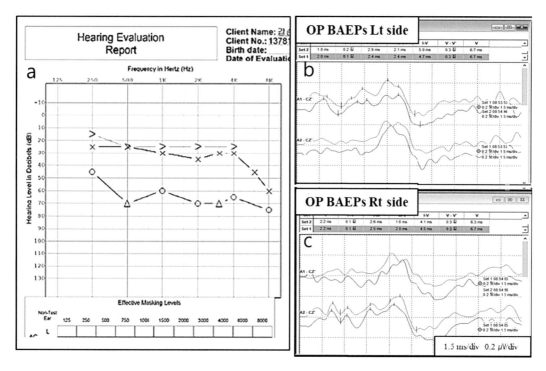

Fig. 8.9 Preoperative pure tone audiometry (**a**), preoperative BAEPs (**b**), intraoperative BAEPs (**c**)

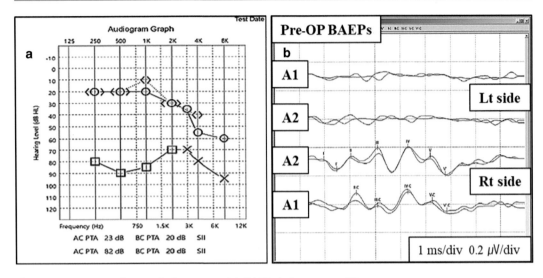

Fig. 8.10 Pure tone audiometry before surgery (**a**), BAEPs before surgery (**b**)

poor listening to a specific frequency band due to sensorineural hearing loss. And it is thought that the BAEPs wave induced by the auditory nerve can be measured as normal because the auditory nerve is generally excited by sound stimulation.

8.1.4.1 Both-Side High-Frequency Sensory Neural Hearing Loss Patient by Noise Exposure

Patients with Lt. HFS M/55 and had high-frequency hearing loss due to noise exposure before surgery (Fig. 8.11a). In the preoperative BAEPs test, the amplitude of wave V on the left, where high-frequency hearing loss was a little more severe, was measured. It is thought that the patient's cooperation during the examination was not smooth (Fig. 8.11b), and there was no difference between left and right in the BAEPs waveform during surgery (Fig. 8.11c).

It is believed that high-frequency hearing loss due to noise exposure does not have a significant effect on the waveform of BAEPs.

8.1.4.2 Left-Side Chronic Mesenteritis Patient

A patient with Rt. HFS F/66 who had otitis media in his left ear before surgery and had high-

frequency hearing loss on both sides (Fig. 8.12a, b). In the BAEPs during surgery, the amplitude of the wave V on the left side with otitis media was largely measured (Fig. 8.12c).

Partial high-frequency hearing loss due to otitis media is not considered to have a significant effect on the waveform of BAEPs.

8.2 The Relationship Between PTA and BAEPs in Cerebellopontine Angle Tumor Patients

8.2.1 Case of Left-Side Small-Sized Tumor and Normal Hearing Patient

A patient with Lt. meningioma F/69 complained of trigeminal neuralgia in the Lt side V2 area. He had no hearing problems before surgery (Fig. 8.13a). It is a preoperative MRI picture and a small-sized tumor is seen (Fig. 8.13b), and there was no difference in left and right of BAEPs waveform during surgery (Fig. 8.13c).

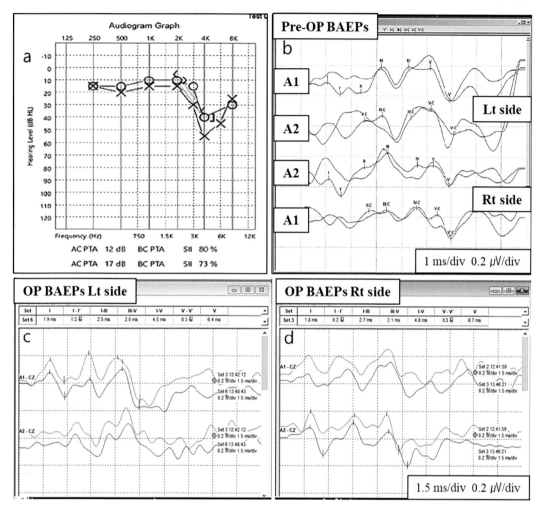

Fig. 8.11 Preoperative pure tone audiometry (**a**), preoperative BAEPs (**b**), intraoperative BAEPs (**c**, **d**)

8.2.2 Case of Right-Side Middle-Size Tumor and High-Frequency Hearing Loss Patient

A patient with Rt. vestibular schwannoma F/37 had a slight tinnitus and weak high-frequency hearing loss on the right side (Fig. 8.14a). It is a preoperative MRI image, and a small tumor of 20.98 mm size is seen (Fig. 8.14b). During the surgery, the BAEPs waveform was observed to extend the wave V latency by 2.3 ms and decrease the amplitude by 0.2 μV on the right side compared to the left (Fig. 8.14c, d).

8.2.3 Case of Right-Side Middle-Size Tumor and High-Frequency Hearing Loss Patient

A patient with Rt. meningioma F/65 had moderate high-frequency hearing loss on the right

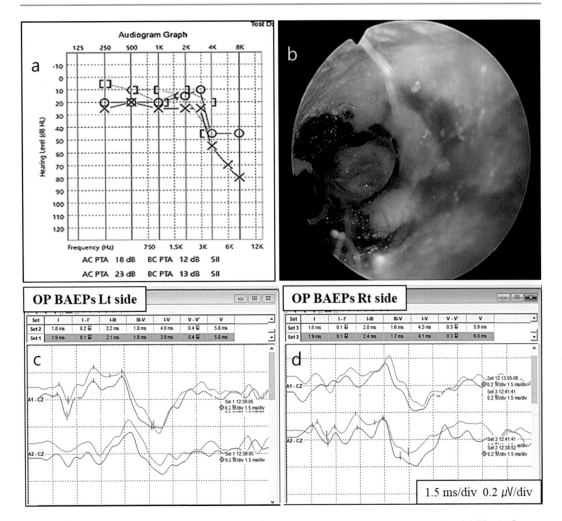

Fig. 8.12 Preoperative pure tone audiometry (**a**), preoperative tympanic picture (**b**), intraoperative BAEPs (**c**, **d**)

side (Fig. 8.15a). This is a preoperative MRI picture, and a small tumor larger than 30 mm is seen (Fig. 8.15b). During the operation, the BAEPs waveform was not measured compared to the patient's right hearing loss slightly (Fig. 8.15c).

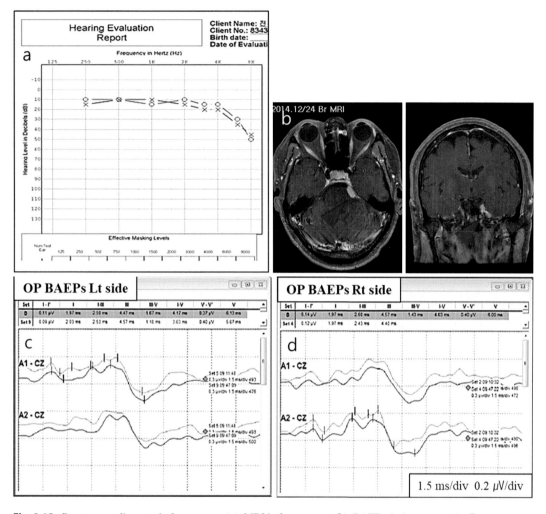

Fig. 8.13 Pure tone audiometry before surgery (**a**), MRI before surgery (**b**), BAEPs during surgery (**c, d**)

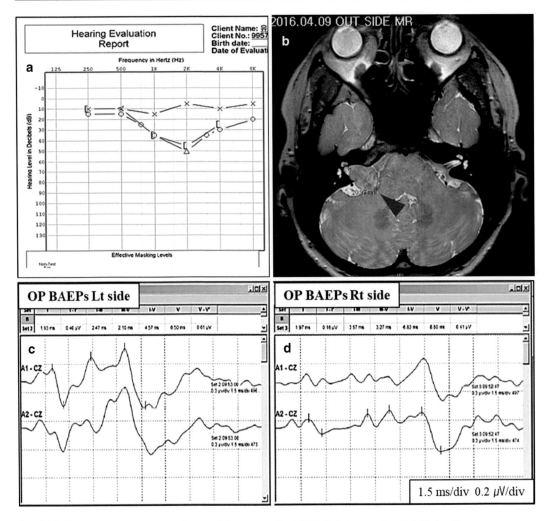

Fig. 8.14 Preoperative pure tone audiometry (**a**), preoperative MRI (**b**), intraoperative BAEPs (**c, d**)

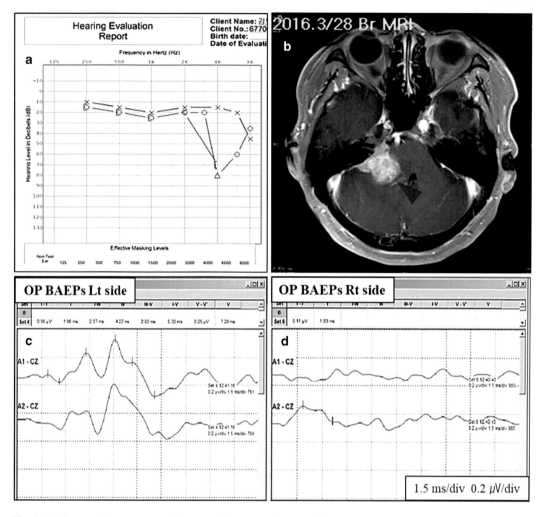

Fig. 8.15   Preoperative pure tone audiometry (**a**), preoperative MRI (**b**), intraoperative BAEPs (**c, d**)

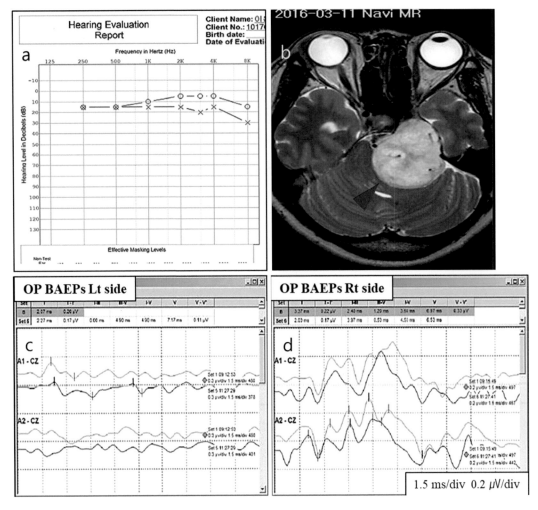

Fig. 8.16 Preoperative pure tone audiometry (**a**), preoperative MRI (**b**), intraoperative BAEPs (**c, d**)

8.2.4 Case of Left-Side Big Size Tumor and Normal Hearing Patient

A patient with Lt. trigeminal schwannoma F/51 had facial pain on the left side and very mild high-frequency hearing loss (Fig. 8.16a). It is a preoperative MRI picture, and a small tumor larger than 60 mm is seen (Fig. 8.16b). During surgery, the BAEPs waveform was not measured compared to the patient's left hearing loss slightly (Fig. 8.16c).

8.3 Conclusion

BAEPs wave V latency delay was observed in the case of severe hearing loss with conductive hear-

ing loss starting from 60 dB in the high-frequency region. Patients with conductive hearing loss and sensorineural hearing loss did not affect the BAEPs waveform even if they were not able to hear a little in the high-frequency range. However, patients with hearing loss due to brain tumors may affect the BAEPs waveform, and even if the patient's hearing is subjectively normal, the BAEPs waveform may not be measured because the excitement of the auditory nerve by sound stimulation is not smoothly transmitted. Evoked potentials must have a basic function that can be evoked by stimulation.

Evoked potentials, we think, should have a basic function that can be evoked by stimulation; therefore when the nerve is affected by the tumor, the nerve function exists, but cannot be evoked by the simulation, so the BAEPs waveform does not form.

References

1. American Academy of Otolaryngology-Head and Neck Surgery Foundation I. Committee on hearing and equilibrium guidelines for the evaluation of results of treatment of conductive hearing loss. Otolaryngol Head Neck Surg. 1995 Sep;113(3):186–7. https://doi.org/10.1016/S0194-5998(95)70103-6.

2. American Academy of Otolaryngology-Head and Neck Surgery Foundation I. Committee on Hearing and equilibrium guidelines for the evaluation of hearing preservation in acoustic neuroma (vestibular schwannoma). Otolaryngol Head Neck Surg. 1995 Sep;113(3):179–80. https://doi.org/10.1016/S0194-5998(95)70101-X.

Printed by Printforce, the Netherlands